Married to **FIBRO**

Tina Marie Birkhoff

Married to Fibro

Cover Design and Page Design: Alexis Kristen Birkhoff
Editing: Karla Sorenson
Author's photo is personal property.

The advice and strategies contained herein may not be suitable for every situation. Procedures, suggestions and ideas are not intended to be a substitute for professional consult or consultation with your physician. The author or publisher shall not be responsible or liable for any loss or damage allegedly arising from any information or suggestions in this book. The fact that an organization or website is referred to in this book as a citation and/or a potential source of further information does not mean that the author or publisher endorses the information the organization or website may provide. Readers need be aware that internet websites listed in this work may have changed or disappeared between when this book was written and when it was read.

ISBN-13: 978-1539346746
ISBN-10: 1539346749
Printed in the United States of America

Dedication

To My Husband,
As the journey continues
I love you more every day.

Tina

Table of Contents

Introduction

Over 5 million people have been diagnosed with Fibromyalgia in the United States alone. This does not include those who silently suffer without a clarification of what or why they are challenged by debilitating pain. I can only relay what I see and what I experience. I am the wife of a man with Fibromyalgia. Only 10% of people diagnosed with fibro are men. That leaves 90% of those out there to be moms, wives, daughters, sisters, grandmothers, and girlfriends with fibromyalgia, chronic pain and fatigue.

We are the support systems for these loved ones when they are in their times of great pain and suffer horribly. I have lived with fibro in my house for almost two decades. Several of my friends have fibro and look for support with little or no success outside their friend circle. I've seen the frustration, sadness, lost hope and despair that affects the sufferer, the spouse, and the rest of the family. We, the family and friends, are a silent group hurting on the inside but saying very little. There have not been systems of support for those of us on this side of fibromyalgia. Married to Fibro is the awareness and recognition of the need for that support. I have written this for you. Through my words in Married to Fibro I support you and I am happy to share with you.

With 18 years of experience Married to Fibro is a book of hope, education, and support. There is hope and life after the diagnosis of Fibromyalgia. Life does continue forward and I am proof! Using the best-of times and not-so-fun times, I will show you day-to-day living with pain and uncertainty. Today is the day you and your loved ones start living a new life. Dive into my life, my findings and new-found hope. You will learn more about the disease and how to support your loved one who has chronic pain and fatigue. But more than that, I hope to encourage you to be a better, stronger, more joyful you in the light of supporting someone with Fibromyalgia.

In The Beginning

What would be the marketable value of a crystal ball if it really worked? Would someone really want a glimmer of what is to come if it was not something they were expecting? Would a peek into the future twenty years give you answers you expect or surprises you would rather not have known? Would it help you appreciate what you have today or mourn the loss of what was missing tomorrow?

When I first met Brent, he would joke, "One day I am going to have llamas." As a farm girl myself knowing this college-going young man had professional plans for his future, I had convinced myself I was not going to be moving back onto a farm anytime in the future. Well, that was one of many premonitions that proves I am not a fortune teller. But more about that later.

Seeing my husband's physical health deteriorate before my eyes is one of those times in my life that I am glad a crystal ball does not work. Although being prepared for the unknown would have been helpful, the anxiety of knowing the severity of his pain and fear would have been too great for me. If I would have known of his pain years in advance, I probably would have developed a very dysfunctional relationship with him, keeping him sheltered and safe from his inevitable future. The rest of the family would have been taken down in this self-controlled dysfunction as well. I learned something about myself in the moment of decision-making without that crystal ball. I am good in emergency situations. I can get organized quickly, and I cut out the unnecessary elements life throws my way in all of the confusion.

Days before diagnosis had become increasingly frustrating as the winter that year was coming to a close. Usually we would be planning a to-do list of projects to accomplish, people to see, places to go for the upcoming warmer months. I felt as though my husband, Brent, was disappearing from the picture. His interest in the family, work, his own life, and living in general had begun to fade.[1] His health was suffering also. He spent more and more time sleeping and lying on the couch. Seldom was he positive about anything more than what he had to eat that day. And often that didn't please him. What was happening to this man who once stood strong at the forefront of this family?

Prior to any signs of a possible illness, Brent was a successful businessman. We owned our third home in five years and we thought we were living the American dream. Brent was working a job he loved. Life was moving quickly, and even though there were times I was overwhelmed, Brent was in his glory. Remember that llama farm? We had two beautiful girls, a small hobby farm, and a few animals. Before having children, I had a good-paying job in Chicago. Now, I had my girls and gardens that replaced my career. I was an at–home mom. I too enjoyed the quiet farm life when it was not in chaos.

Three years into our farm life, Brent had not been himself for several months, and his increasing lack of interest in even the simplest of tasks was wearing on me. One evening after I settled the girls down for bed, Brent informed me that his chest had been bothering him, he had numbness in his left arm all day, and he felt it was getting worse. He also had no desire to have it checked. Being conservative with health issues because of cost was one thing. This was not one of those times and I was not going to let him sit and wait it out. After quietly packing an activity bag for the girls (5 and 7 years old) and putting their sleeping bags by the door, I convinced Brent that a visit to the E.R. was a must. Was this a heart attack?!

There was a barrage of doctors' visits that followed in the next few months. It was not a heart attack or any cardiovascular issues at all. This was bittersweet knowing what it was not. Now what was it? The results were all inconclusive at best. After a few months and many tests and professionals later, an upper GI was performed.

As we sat in the recovery area, the doctor gave us his professional opinion, "Take this little purple pill daily, and in a week you'll feel like a new man." I almost scoffed at him. The doctor declared all of his symptoms were from acid reflux disease! This was the diagnosis? Not for a moment did we believe that the little purple pill would relieve all the symptoms he was experiencing. His floating joint pain, the chest pains, abdominal and intestinal pain, debilitating fatigue, the headaches, light headedness, the numbness in his hands, the restless leg kicking at night and the overall pain that kept this over-achiever home from work could not be that easily cured. He filled the prescription and followed the instructions carefully with limited hope. That expensive little pill did nothing. No surprise!

Through the encouragement of a friend who had just gone through his own emergency situation and my strong encouragement, we took an emergency trip to The Mayo Clinic in Rochester, Minnesota. Within a few hours we had an overnight stay planned, a baby-sitter, and no appointment at the clinic. The lack of an appointment didn't matter. We still set off to find what we prayed would not be an expensive adventure to nowhere or worse, a terminal diagnosis. We stayed three days for the first round of tests. The Mayo Clinic is thorough and leaves no doubt when a diagnosis is determined. They made sure it was not a long list of possibilities. We found them to be an incredible institution of research and knowledge. After a week and a half and thousands of dollars in test and blood work, I was with Brent to hear his diagnosis. The doctor said he had Fibromyalgia. Now that we had a name, what was it?

Fibro what?

The doctor visits at the Mayo Clinic had been a series of hurry-up-and-wait appointments. We were filling cancelled slots and sitting in the hotel room awaiting another appointment. I had traded my bi-annual weekend get-away, a mom's conference, for a sheet of paper with dates and times of appointments I would walk to with Brent. We walked away from the last one of the week relieved and baffled. He even spent a second week alone at the clinic having more tests for verification of a diagnosis. After Brent went through 15 separate exams, stress tests, and blood draws we were given one word, Fibromyalgia. With silent relief we walked the underground walkways of the Mayo Clinic which attaches to all of the surrounding hotels and shops. There was a Barnes and Noble in the underground walkway system, they knew of this odd disease as I saw the window display featuring a medical book about Fibromyalgia.

Today, I would still choose to support Brent, but at the time it was hard to not feel extended frustration. My refueling, relaxing, and reconnecting to life was supposed to happen during this weekend with my friends. I know he appreciated my support but I am not sure he understood the sacrifice. I know he needed me there. The week after his diagnosis, he returned alone for the follow-up appointments. The sessions walked the patient through how to continue living with this disease. Brent was lonely and missing my companionship as he returned to his room, but his exhaustion had him asleep as soon as his head hit the pillow. I was also feeling lonely, but for different reasons. My husband was never going to be the same.[2] Where was the session for the spouse?

Fibromyalgia is characterized by stiffness and achy body pain in soft tissues such as muscles, tendons, and ligaments. It is a wide-spread pain throughout the body. Abdominal pain, constipation and diarrhea difficulties are also symptoms of fibro. Many patients are seen for arthritic symptoms, numbness in extremities, debilitating fatigue, and migraines on a regular basis. Think about the last time you had the stomach flu. The day after suffering the worst of the virus one feels achy, sore, slow, and overall not well. That is the general description of a fibro sufferer on a daily basis.

This all looks so clean cut in the print of a book. Yes, he suffered from that, check, and that, check. But Brent suffered from all of this. Our insurance would cover eighty percent of his Mayo Clinic visit and none of the hotel or dining expenses. This was a big financial burden for us. There wasn't a chapter in the books about this. Being thrifty, I actually brought ready-to-eat dinners for our daily meals to save some money. There are around 5 million Americans affected by Fibromyalgia.[3] That is a lot of households making a large emotional and physical contribution to something so vague.

There are no known causes for Fibromyalgia that have been documented but there are a few suspicions. A severe accident at a stressful time in a person's life has been associated with the start of fibro symptoms for some sufferers. Others associate it with the results of a harsh illness, a severe infection, or the antibiotics used to cure the illness, such as drugs in the fluoroquinolone family like ciprofloxacin, "Cipro".[4] Brent had been treated with this drug more than once when he was in his early twenties. Researchers have also added hormonal changes to the extended list of possible fibro starters. This does give one reason to question if any of these could be the culprit.

Brent was on a trip to Florida when he felt he was coming down with the flu. Prior to this incident he had felt healthy with no outstanding unusual issues. Not long into the trip, he called home and said he felt like he'd been hit by a train. He had nausea and dizziness throughout the day and was exhausted. For the next several weeks he felt these symptoms and more issues accumulating. Many patients have no preceding conditions whatsoever before the symptoms of fibro set in. They just want an answer for why they have it.

No two people's pain is the same with fibro sufferers. This is one of the most confusing and frustrating issues with Fibromyalgia. Pain may occur for some on a constant basis, and for another it floats and varies, while others have symptoms that look very much like other illnesses. Fibromyalgia has several illnesses that mimic the same symptoms and need attention by a professional. Self-diagnosing fibro is not advised. With advertising barraging us daily, this is not hard to do. Hypothyroidism, Lupus, Lyme disease, and Interstitial cystitis are conditions that should not go unattended for fear of quickly becoming worse. Irritable bowel syndrome (IBS), sleep apnea, and TMJ problems are all conditions with varying degrees of symptoms and problems. Brent's fibro combines some symptoms of several ailments like his roaming pain is a symptom of Lyme disease. He has sleep difficulty similar to sleep apnea and IBS difficulties just to name a few. Add to these frightening ailments like headaches, blurred vision and numbness in his fingers, which mimic brain disorders.

To complicate matters, many people discontinue advanced diagnosis because a doctor may tell them their symptoms are simply stress related and recommend a counselor. So many of the doctors Brent saw didn't even believe Fibromyalgia was a valid disease. The pain and suffering is very real even though the sufferers look completely healthy. Hearing that it is all in their head is very degrading and humiliating. The sufferer will often go back into their cave of pain and suffer alone, quietly, while family members wonder where their loved one has disappeared.

With every person comes a different set of conditions and ailments. To add to the complexity, every person has a different reaction to the treatment and medications. Depending on the treatment, some have varying degrees of alleviation to the pain and some no relief at all. My cupboard started to look like a mini pharmacy. I never thought I'd experience that at 40. Is it any wonder why so many doubt their symptoms and diagnosis? Brent went through multiple medications. Some made him sick, some caused weight gain, and some did nothing at all.

Pharmaceuticals are not the only option for relief to fibro pain. Massage, yoga, acupuncture, and dietary change have been known to help some sufferers. Brent goes to a masseuse on a monthly basis, in addition to a few medications, exercise, a vitamin regiment, and a healthy diet.

With all these inconsistencies, the fibro sufferer has yet another symptom to battle, and that is depression. Many sufferers have never been diagnosed with depression before fibro. So, why after? Being in constant pain, not feeling as one felt years ago, and having to take medication that may be alleviating only some of the symptoms day after day takes a toll on ones psyche.

This I know for sure. With the right doctor and the proper treatment, life can return to a pleasant, livable condition with only a few alterations. The reality is that it may take some financial strain to find the right treatment but it is not impossible, and if the treatment is not working, it is time to move on to someone else who can help.

As a kid, I remember my brothers and I would show off our "war wounds" of play as though they were rewards. When asked "Aw man, does it hurt?" with my arm in a cast, I'd say, "Nah, it only hurts when…" We seemed indestructible. Our nervous system is uniquely designed to alert us of pain through millions of small nerves. So, what is different in a person with fibro from those of us without the disease? Researchers have found that fibro patients have an elevated level of Substance P, three times higher than people without the condition. Substance P is found in the spinal cord and is responsible for sending pain messages from the body to the brain. Hence, people with fibro feel pain three times greater than those without.

To add another factor to the pain a person with fibro feels, they have a decreased amount of serotonin in their system. Serotonin tells the body the pain they feel really isn't as bad as it appears. I can endure a painful toe stub on the sofa leg much more than Brent can. My pain is evident and unpleasant but Brent's pain is excruciating and long lasting.

Brent and I started riding our bikes for exercise a few years ago. Usually it takes several weeks to work up to a lengthy ride on the open road rather than on the smooth flat bike path. Brent has complained of tail bone pain after riding. Normally, the body will build up muscle and tissue to alleviate the pain. I asked Brent how long it will take for that pain to go away. He said it will be there the entire riding season. He endures the pain knowing the riding benefits are greater than the consequences of not exercising. His body regenerates muscle and tissue much differently than mine.

Our bodies heal when we sleep. It is no coincidence then why people sleep so much more when they are sick. The body is demanding healing time. Typically an uninterrupted 8-hour sleep is recommended for a healthy lifestyle. The typical Fibro person will feel like they may be getting the right amount of sleep but the body isn't performing a healthy sleep cycle. During the deepest sleep, the REM period of sleep, the body regenerates cell tissue that replaces weak and injured cells. This is a self-healing system. The body keeps itself healthy when we get proper amounts of sleep. Sleep deprivation is also a symptom and a contributor to Fibro. Typically, fibro sufferers do not get enough REM sleep; therefore, a lack of cell regeneration in deep muscle tissue creates heightened sensitivity to pain.[5] The lack of REM sleep creates a vicious cycle where the body cannot regenerate muscle tissue to eliminate the pain, which enhances the pain, creating exhaustion during the day, and a craving for more sleep.

Stephanie, our first born child, is a beautiful flute player. When she entered into high school, she enthusiastically joined marching band. We as proud parents dedicated our Friday nights and weekends to cheering her band on throughout the weeks of competition. Little did we know that although the season was only six weeks long, it often concluded in the late hours of the night or started in the early hours of the morning, and on some weekends there were both early mornings and late nights. Brent would not get his required amount of sleep and felt completely wrung out. He had so little energy, he started to rely on a prescription drug to keep him awake. Then at night, when we got home, he'd take a medication to help him sleep. It wasn't long before I questioned his motives. I didn't understand why the need for prescription drugs that battled each other. I am not a medication taker. If I can go without, I do. My concern went far deeper than my habits.

Brent did not want to listen to his body and take a break from some activity at home so he could be rested for the band competitions or take a night off from competitions. He needed to prioritize his desires and activities. It is known that medical interns take this same prescription to get them through their long hours in medical school, so the drug is considered safe. But Brent did stop taking the "awake" prescription mostly due to my concerns. He has tried some energy drinks but found they didn't work for him and he didn't like the taste. Ultimately, he just needs a nap or a later morning alarm. Band is officially over now and our flautist graduated, so our band competitions are a thing of the past. I hope a lesson has been learned as well. Take care of getting enough sleep first and medicate only the uncontrollable issues.

We are used to Brent going to bed like clock-work. At 8:50 p.m. he drinks his cocktail of magnesium and vitamin D with a sleep aid, kisses each of us goodnight and proceeds up the "wooden hill." We hear him turn out the light at 9:20 until 4:50 a.m. Ours is a quiet home. We like it that way or we've grown accustomed to it that way. I'm not sure how to determine which one it is. If the girls were out past 9:00 p.m., I was the parent that stayed up for their late arrival or the necessary pick up. He seldom sees 10:00 p.m. It was at times a sacrifice for me. I got tired. I would have liked the option to go to bed early. However, I don't have pain so I waited up awhile. I didn't suffer memory loss or debilitating fatigue if I had to pick someone up after hours. This was one of my silent contributions to his health that I know would eventually conclude when our youngest went to college.

Common symptoms of Fibromyalgia

Why is Fibromyalgia so difficult to diagnosis? Why has it created such a flurry of concern and interest without a solid diagnosis? Many sufferers float from one doctor to another without much relief from the pain and exhaustion. They go through their day-to-day routine looking healthy and feeling anything but that internally. Home and work routines are greatly disrupted by the pain, fatigue, and other symptoms that come with fibro. The pain can actually get debilitating enough to cause the sufferer to not be able to work or accomplish simple daily routines.

Here are the most common symptoms that occur in someone with fibro. However, not everyone with fibro suffers from every one of these symptoms nor is every symptom listed due to the fact that some symptoms are more individualistic and not commonly considered an issue for diagnosis.

Widespread pain – Although Brent states he has pain in only one or two areas of his body, he often would admit to a low grade pain throughout his entire body. After strenuous activity he can also have pain that lasts for a long period of time and is in an area that is not normally afflicted. For some people it is constant and for others it is sporadic. There are 18 possible tender points (nine on one side of the body, nine on the other). When light pressure is applied, fibro patients feel tremendous pain. To be diagnosed one must have pain for at least three documented, consecutive months and in 11 of the 18 tender points affected.[6]

Headaches – The phrase "migraine headache" has become a description used for a severe headache that can be eased or eliminated with medication. Most fibro headaches are not of a migraine caliber, but with all the other pain circulating around their body, the head is the last desirable place to have pain. Headaches for the fibro patient are often a symptom that is not easily relieved with common medication. The high level of exhaustion creates many symptoms, including visual changes and eye pain.[7] Patients often request different prescription medications and complain that the pain lasts days without much relief.

IBS (Irritable Bowel Syndrome) - Think about trying to function from one day to another without knowing if you'll spend it running to the bathroom or wishing you could once you get there. Stomach pain, abdominal discomfort, and embarrassing physical conditions are a prominent symptom of many fibro sufferers. One day it can be in the form of constipation and the next day diarrhea. The discomfort and unknown conditions from day to day often are more detrimental to the persons' activities than the fibro pain itself.

Fibro Fog – A typical Friday in our home is quite humorous if one were watching from the sidelines. I believe in the family eating together as often as possible. I usually make meals from scratch and try to make them as healthy as possible. As the girls filled us in on their school happenings and what their weekend would hold, we often found Brent staring into space. One of the girls inevitably would call out, "Hellloooo… Earth to dad!" He usually snapped to and asked what we were talking about. We would all laugh and start the conversation over only in a much shorter version. Similar to walking in a daze, many patients experience a condition that can create confusion and memory lapses. Staring into space, mixing up words, and having difficulty concentrating are characteristics of the fog which is caused by debilitating fatigue. After his long complex week at work it is no surprise that fatigue is what he is feeling.

The Drops – Friday's fatigue is also met with the usual utensil drop and an occasional spill. When the girls were toddlers, it was common to have items spilt or dropped on the floor. Now we accept that it is the end of the week and Brent will have the expected "dropsies." Muscles and joints become tired and dropping things for no reason is very common at the end of a long week for fibro patients.

Tingling hands and feet – Imagine having the feeling of your hands going to sleep, and the tingling that comes many times in a day or constantly throughout the day. Many fibro patients say they have experienced numbness, tingling, or burning. While mostly in their hands or feet, some experience it in other parts of the body as well. This is sometimes mistaken as carpal tunnel syndrome or even multiple sclerosis and unnecessary medications are prescribed or surgery is performed.[8]

Restless Leg Syndrome – More than fifty percent of us spouses get to experience this from across the bed at night, those little kicks right before Brent falls asleep and often after. Although these symptoms come and go, they occur mostly at night. Restless leg syndrome is part of the sleep deprivation that the fibro sufferer experiences. Whether it is from an illness, not being able to relax into sleep, or being overly exhausted and unable sleep, all are causes and symptoms for sleep disruption.

Climate Sensitivities – We love visiting relatives in Colorado. Many of our vacations were spent there and not at Disney World. The number one reason is that Brent has no fibro pain when we visit there. Now, I am not eliminating the fact that Brent is not under the everyday stresses of work and the routine that comes with it. An increased sensitivity to light, barometric pressure, temperature changes, dampness, humidity, and drafts are all part of the hypersensitivity of the nervous system. Colorado is a dry environment, with a lot of sun and a more constant temperature than Wisconsin. There is also a great deal of beautiful terrain to walk for pleasure doubling as exercise.

Stress – He who lives without stress is incredibly fortunate. Brent leaves the care of the house to me while he works very hard at his job in the textile industry. I'd like to say I make homeownership easy for him, but that would not be true. Every-day maintenance and bills do their fair share of giving stress. Although stress is a contributing factor to illness, it is especially difficult for fibro patients. The biggest culprits are not necessarily the major stress factors in our lives but the annoying day-to-day hassles that affect chronic pain.

Sleeplessness – Sleep apnea, insomnia, restless leg syndrome and unrested sleep are all difficulties a person with fibro may experience. Professional sleep studies have shown that not having a television in the bedroom, destressing, eliminating caffeinated beverages after supper, keeping pets out of the bedroom and reducing afternoon naps are all part of the "get a better night's sleep" list.[9] Before Brent had a sleep aide, he was often found reading in the living room in the middle the night to induce sleep. One of the major contributing factors to fibro chronic pain is lack of deep sleep. The body regenerates cell tissue while sleeping, repairing and restoring muscle tissue. Fibro sufferers do not get into a deep sleep (REM, Rapid Eye Movement) that allows the cell regeneration to occur.

Anxiety – How much pain will I be in tomorrow? Will I be able to accomplish all I desire? When will I feel relatively healthy and pain free? Phrases like these fill the mind of a fibro sufferer. Anxiety can appear to be a "state of mind" for those with fibro. But it is a heightened issue for some fibro sufferers. Anxiety can escalate other symptoms based on the stress it creates.

Depression – With constant aches and unwanted pain, being positive is very difficult for a fibro sufferer. I have a very good friend with fibro. From the outside she appears joyful and happy. Sit down with her for a cup of coffee at the end of a busy week and I get an entirely different view of my friend's life. She is in pain. She feels she is not getting things done around her house due to her exhaustion, while her family does not understand her frustration or feelings of being overwhelmed. Brent too slows down at the end of a busy week and often feels very overwhelmed. He questions how he will be able to get his weekend to-do list done. When will he get time to relax? Often triggered by ongoing stress, depression causes changes in mood. Feelings of sadness, anxiety, and being down only complicate the physical symptoms of fibro. More pain, more stress, more sadness, more depression, more stress, more pain. The cycle continues if the depression is not confronted.

What Fibromyalgia Is NOT

The thought of having chronic pain sounds like a form of torture, and to fibromyalgia sufferers it can be. From no cause, no cure and very little consistencies in a diagnosis to learn from they feel lost and often alone. On the plus side, for those of us loved ones, there is hope.

Not all in the head - One of the first visits my husband had with his general practitioner after being diagnosed with fibro was an eye opener. The doctor told Brent he didn't believe in Fibro, that it was a "cliché" phrase for "I don't know what is causing you pain," and he felt it was all in Brent's head. We were told that doctor has since changed his mind. However, at that moment my husband felt completely shut off from his ability to feel safe with and trusted by this physician. He spent several years and many office visits trying to find the right doctor. One doctor felt multiple medications were needed; few of them helped alleviate pain, and many left a trail of nasty side effects. Another doctor wanted to treat every symptom with a separate remedy. Yet another wanted him to go on a special diet, exercise routine, and come back for visits and blood work often. The doctors all tried to help, but he felt few were listening to him and his needs.[10] He did find a few doctors he trusted greatly and a comfortable form of pain treatment. Yes, stress is in your head and in our lives. But the pain is very real and very much in the body.

Not the end – By the time Brent was diagnosed with fibro we were living in our third purchased house. We hate the buying and selling of homes, but the adventure of making this new residence our home was quite thrilling for us. Trying to sell any house we called home has been far from pleasurable. The first realtor we hired for our second house, the Victorian, went through an inspection with our buyer and exclaimed the house was a standing fire hazard, scaring the buyer away. Days later a professional electrician declared the property completely safe. Those few days of waiting for the professional to visit were horrible. We had a bridge loan on another property, a beautiful 18 acre farm. What were we going to do if we could not sell this house? Thankfully, the stress and anxiety were wasted time and energy. With a new realtor and a positive outlook, we sold the house in a matter of weeks.

The stress of finding a diagnosis for fibro can feel very much the same. This is not a life-threatening disease. However, it is life altering. Our minds' imagined a diagnosis such as cancer or some other deadly disease before Brent finally visited the Mayo Clinic. There was so much time wasted on the stress and anxiety of what he could have, that we lost focus on living life. Now that we are on the other side of diagnosis, we know it is not an end but just a beginning of an altered lifestyle. Getting to bed earlier, exercising more frequently, and eating a healthy diet with very limited carbohydrates, lots of water, and plenty of fruits and vegetables have improved fibro symptoms and the entire family's health. To add to those advantages, a healthier lifestyle also lowers stress and heightens endorphins that help improve one's overall outlook on life and eliminate pain.

Nowhere to turn – One of Brent's dreams from childhood was to own a llama farm. As the wife on the farm, I felt it my responsibility to care for the creatures when Brent worked. I am not a fan of animals larger than a cat. If I don't feel capable of controlling their environment, I don't want to be a part of it. Brent worked an hour from home and seldom could get off work at a drop of a hat if I had a "farm emergency." Part of the farming was the breeding of the llamas so we owned a male llama. He was not the kindest creature. I don't think he would have done physical harm to a person but his spitting and aggression were highly intimidating. As with most llamas he always tested the fence. He wanted to be in with the girls, and he'd do whatever it would take to get there. As was the case when my 7 year old got off the bus announcing he was in the ditch trying to get into the other pasture. In trying to capture and halter him, I unfortunately chased him across the road into the neighbor's field. What a predicament! My youngest had little fear of larger animals. She was a big helper. She haltered up a female while I set up a mobile pen unit and lured him in with his girlfriend's beauty. He had nowhere to go except to do as I commanded. The girlfriend went back to her pasture and he was tethered to a tree to eat grass until the fence could be checked and Brent could get home.

Being diagnosed with an incurable disease can feel a lot like that male llama's life. He wanted something different. He wanted out of his situation. Being penned up is not the most fun way of living life but it is the most safe. As of now, there is no cure for fibro. There are more studies being done to find medication to help alleviate the pain as quickly as chemists can develop them. As a spouse, we can offer support and compassion during times of need. Having a positive attitude and a listening ear does wonders too. Often the person in pain just needs to be heard. We cannot heal them but we can be present to them. There are many Fibromyalgia support groups also. Calling your local hospital may help locate the nearest one.

The blame game – I am an oldest child. If you check the definition of "the first born child syndrome," I may be mentioned. There were only 4 children in my family but I felt responsible for all of us. My mother continuously reminded me that I was not responsible for everyone and everything. Actually, she may have said, "Mind your own business" or "You are not the mother." Either would have been appropriate for "Little Miss Bossy" me. Ironically, Brent is also a first born. This has made for some very interesting family decision-making. After having the girls, I found my sense of responsibility losing its boundaries. Some of the smallest issues felt like they were my fault. I took it on as my issue to resolve. Brent being "Mr. Type A" and a first born tends to point out when things are not quite perfect. Magazines that may be sitting on a coffee table unattended, broccoli that was served as more stumps than florets, children that were whiny instead of happy are all examples of what might be pointed out. I felt responsible to correct the issues. After a while I began predicting what he would point out next. This really became an issue for me. I needed to let go of the small stuff and focus on the real issues at hand. Why was Brent so driven to perfection? Could I really please this drive? I was not the cause of his disappointment; therefore, I was not responsible for the resolution. Yes, a magazine or two are on the coffee table, but no, my broccoli is not full of stumps.

Feeling responsible for more than me was a part of my life. I even went as far as feeling responsible for others' happiness. Were others comfortable? Did they need something from me even if it meant me sacrificing something of myself? I have learned the term "co-dependent." I was co-dependent. I gave more of myself to others and not enough to take care of my own immediate needs; this included Brent's overall health and his pain.

There is no one at fault for the pain a fibro person feels. It is important to know that even though it may feel like you get the wrong end of the stick, and you may be the one getting the brunt of the negative emotions, you are not causing the pain. Often times those in pain unload on the ones they love the most. They know they can trust that you will continue to love them. This does not make their emotional dump on you okay. They need to find another outlet or put their feelings in perspective. We family members and spouses need not allow their poor behavior either. We need to express when they are out of line or seem unusually angry or emotional. Again, just listen. You can't fix it, so don't take it on.

The gene pool - Fibromyalgia is not contagious. It cannot be caught, contracted, or passed on physically. However, some research says it can be passed on through heredity in the gene pool and familial behaviors.[11] Brent's aunt suffered from fibro for many years before he was diagnosed. We did not know she had it because she suffered silently. We love his aunt. She is so active and a real go-getter. One would never know she has fibro by looking at her. She is high energy, sometimes to a fault. Taking time to relax comes hard when there are people to visit, places to be, things to do. Brent has the same behavior as his aunt. Is it DNA or behaviorally influenced for Brent? Science and psychology have shown inconclusive studies. What is known is that if one member of a family has fibro then there probably could be another. Knowing that the symptoms are stress enhanced can teach us that if we show our children proper stress relief and stress management it could considerably lessen their possibility of suffering from Fibro.

A happily ever-after – No sugar coating here. Brent and I have had some really trying times. He finds it humorous to tell friends that we have had 7 good years of marriage in the past 25. Ouch! I'm not counting. There will be good days and there will be bad ones. I just hope there are more good, great, and wonderful days than not so great days. Our lifestyles are very different. He is a

> very hard working executive. I am a dreamer and an artist. He wants perfection. I want pleasantries. He likes to have collections. I like unique individuality. There have been times that we have both felt living the single life would be much easier than working at the process of marriage but neither one of us wanted the responsibility of being a single parent. We didn't like the idea of shared parenting. So, we worked through the marriage one day at a time. We have put our dreams into plans for our future so we have something to live for and work towards. Working through the process has made us both grow and change for the better.

Life does change after diagnosis. Honestly, life was changing before diagnosis. Communication is tough at times but highly necessary. Forgiveness and healing of emotions are essential. Simplifying life reduces stress and allows one to appreciate the smaller pleasures we often miss. Seeing life from a different vantage point brings situations into perspective and being thankful for something, anything, brings a sense of peace and well-being. Having an appreciation for what we have at this very moment has become a focus. There could be a lot less: less happiness, less family, less time together, less peace, or less of living. Creating less stress and more peace is an overall good and revitalizing habit and can only contribute to better living.

Perfect Perfection

My husband's favorite meal is lasagna. Even though it is not the healthiest meal for a person with fibro to eat, he savors it the few times a year I prepare it for him. I make it from scratch. I love doing small things like making dinners from scratch and keeping our meals as wholesome as possible. When I can, I even harvest my own fruits and vegetables. I know some may find it overwhelming, but I love it. Pasta layered with homegrown vegetables and farm raised meat is a blessing to behold, with a lettuce salad straight from the garden and the dressing made from scratch. To organize such a lovely spread brings me great pleasure.

When I met my husband in college, he was very detail-orientated, very organized, and meticulous. I was attracted to this part of him and many other characteristics he had. He hung his clothes, categorized all in the same direction in his closet, with the same distance between color coordinated hangers. On the other hand, I had a hand-full of hangers, some with more than one item on them, and didn't think twice about what direction the clothes hung. I am conceptual. I like things in their place but that may mean a pile of envelopes by the phone and a few unread magazines on a table. Organized? Yes, but not meticulous.

After doing a little Internet research about personality types it quickly became obvious I was a Type B and my husband a very strong Type A. I actually thought I might see my husband's name under the Type A category. "If you are a Type A personality you are most like Brent Birkhoff." This realization has shown me so many characteristics to who he is and what he craves, desires, and even demands.

We were commuters in our early marriage. Time was precious. Not a minute was spared by Brent. He read newspapers or books on the way into Chicago on the train and usually read or did work on the way home. He always made notes or tore out articles that interested him as he read. I typically slept. My eyes were closed before the train left the station. I commuted until the first child came along, then I became an at-home mom. Two years later, Brent's position in Chicago was changing and an opportunity of greater interest came up in Milwaukee. He lets no moss grow under his feet. We were two weeks post of having our second child and he was changing jobs with a weekend break in between.

Brent was closing up his position in Chicago and I was closing up the house in Geneva, Illinois. Stephanie was two and Alexis was 2 weeks old as I was left to guide movers to what, where, and how to pack our belongings. I was frustrated at the lack of concern Brent had for me and my needs. So much so that when one of the movers challenged me saying they could not remove some screws in our bedroom set to disassemble, it I let them have it. With a nursing child on my breast, I argued with them about their contract obligations and said I could not do the labor the contract said they were going to do. My abrupt emotions were probably harsh but the nursing child caused the men to do whatever I asked of them until they were finished.

For the typical Type A personality, work is more important to them than relationships. Brent's work always came before the family. I thought it noble, disturbing and frustrating. Type As have very high standards and hence have trouble expecting anything less of others than what they would give.[12] I see now that being a new father and having a change in jobs required him to see his income as a form of security. Brent was a true provider and bread winner and I was grateful for that. He had control of life as long as he had the comfort of the paycheck.

We moved to a Milwaukee suburb temporarily. Living in a gray, gloomy, cold, empty apartment with two babies was one of the lowest times in my life. I didn't have a car and often it was so cold and rainy we couldn't go out so a small television with an antenna was our only solace. The majority of our belongings were in a storage unit while Brent went searching for a better living environment for the family. I found this accommodating but frustrating. I was elbow deep in diapers and wanted nothing better than to have a place to call home other than the ant infested place we were in at the time.

Brent's standards were very high when looking for the perfect place. He needed a large place with a nice yard for very little money. His determination and persistence, typical of a Type A, kept the realtors alert. Although we wanted a two-story, the first realtor spent the day showing us ranch style homes. We wanted quiet and safe. The second realtor took us to houses on busy streets and duplexes. Our third realtor finally knew what we were looking for and found our next home. This was an extremely stressful time for the family.

We were in love with a beautiful two-story Victorian at first sight. The large front porch, sturdy columns, gingerbread details and a perfect carriage house in the back. There were enough bedrooms, bathrooms and living space for our family to grow in for many years to come. It was a sturdy house that needed a coat of paint and some tender loving care.

Not until we began remodeling our Victorian house did I really understand the desire Brent had to be so focused on the completed project. A typical Type A personality tends to race with time.[13] There is never enough time and if they don't act now, the moment will never return. After our offer was accepted for the house, we went to work ordering wallpaper, paint, blinds, and drapes. We hadn't even moved in yet! Brent also felt the renovation would take 3 months. Silly of me to think that child-care might wait as I hung wallpaper and painted while Brent was at work. On nights and weekends Brent pitched in to renovate as well. There was a time frame to adhere to. My codependent personality felt responsible to accomplish as much in the home as he might be doing at work even if it meant neglecting my own needs. I was trying to appease his Type A need to race with time and ignore my Type B patient, creative, easy-going desires. The renovation took 6 months on the inside of the house and 3 months on the outside.

We left no space in the house untouched. I am a designer by trade and an artist at heart. Brent and I really wanted this house to look and be the perfect home. We worked tirelessly from the very date of move-in to accomplish this. The third week after moving in, the second floor bathroom fell into the kitchen below. My heart sank! Brent took the challenge head on. After being rejected by the insurance company because they didn't cover "corrosion" we took out a loan. The girls and I moved to my mom's for three weeks and a contractor took over. Brent's Type A personality shined bright here! The stress of a new job, new home, and an expensive remodel must have been tremendous for him. The kitchen and bath, however, were completed in a timely manner and turned out beautifully.

All of the walls and ceilings in this old house were lath and plaster. There were many cracks and loose areas and we had no desire to spend all the time needed for a complete overhaul. In most cases we placed cotton wall covering over the sanded areas and painted. You'd never know there was a dilapidated wall behind the lovely color. I felt very much like those walls. On the outside I was pretty, put together. The girls were happy. We visited the park and YMCA often while silently my mind review what I could get done today so it didn't look like I had done nothing. I was not doing Brent or myself any justice in covering up my true emotions. Inside I was craving rest and recognition. I was a crumbling mess of emotions and desires.

We stayed in that beautifully decorated home for 2 ½ years. Then, Brent got restless for something bigger and better.

Many studies have shown people with Fibromyalgia tend to be a Type A personality like my husband. They tend to be aggressive, ambitious, controlling, business-like, highly competitive, time-conscious, impatient, preoccupied with status, a workaholic, hostile, tightly-wound, detail-orientated, and organized sometimes to a fault. Type A personalities are over achievers, driven, and loyal to the cause, whatever that cause may be. When life requires detail and organization I think Type A people do know how to put it all in a beautiful package. From beginning to end, they have a plan.[14]

We have had our fair share of personality battles of the Type A personality and the Type B. There had been many a quiet night when Brent went into his "cave" to stew on the issues at hand, leaving me with 25,000 words left to express to the dog.

Controlling life to maximize its potential is very dangerous and can easily get out of hand in no time. Control is often times confused with organization. Being organized allows for a mishap and an opening for change. Control has no room for alterations. Expectation, disappointment, and frustration follow control all over. Stress follows right behind.

I love a perfectly clean home. I just hate getting there. Brent loves a perfectly clean home and would keep on us until completion, if I didn't speak up for the rest of us. I have asked for a softer side to cleaning. The house is clean. Bathrooms and kitchen are cleaned weekly bedrooms are picked up as needed but not daily. Carpets are vacuumed and floors swept weekly (sometimes more due to a messy craft) but not daily. Cleanliness may be next to Godliness, but I think being next to my girls watching a movie or reading on the porch is even closer to God. Time is fleeting and children and family will not always be there. He isn't stressed about the cleanliness of the home any longer though. The house will get clean. There is greater peace now for all of us.

Slowly but surely, we are acquiring the ability to communicate together. Communication was not a strong point for either of our families so we didn't learn that art early on. Brent was great at the silent treatment when we were first married. He'd go for days not saying a word to me. I was crushed. I had a tendency to over analyze the situation and wanted to talk about it as soon as it happened. Brent wanted the time to think through the argument and did not want to discuss it at all with me. Once the silent treatment was over, it was normal living as usual without mentioning the situation again. I could not have been more aggravated. How were we going to avoid that issue from happening again if we didn't work it out? His personality type does not like to think there could possibly be something wrong with him. There must be something wrong with everyone else. He's learning to hear me more clearly through my organized, well thought out conversation.

I am by no means perfect. I don't want to be. There is way too much expected of one who is perfect. In knowing Brent's desire for organization I try to keep the house picked up. He is now often heard saying “I am a recovering Type A”. We are also now aware that without communication our stress levels go up. Life continues with or without perfection. However, it runs much more smoothly with communication.

Digging in Deeper

The dream of owning a "Hobby Farm" was alluring because I could grow organic fruits and vegetables, the girls would have room to run and grow, and Brent would perhaps find time to appreciate life and have a few animals. We moved into our three-bedroom house on 18 beautiful acres where we acquired 2 large sheep and several laying hens with the property. As inexperienced animal farmers we did not know the sheep were an aggressive breed and unsafe. The electric fence would not contain them so the girls had to stay inside or very close to the house for safety. One of my first experiences with the escapees was on a warm spring day with the windows wide open while the girls were napping. I was sitting by a window folding laundry enjoying the quiet when "Baaaaaah, Baaaaah," came right from behind me. Mere inches away, the two sheep were watching me fold laundry from outside the window! I nearly lost my heart and the hairs on the back of my neck still stand up remembering it. My first farm job was to get the electric fence up and running in a timely fashion, for there were two llamas on their way, and I didn't need them watching me fold laundry.

The stress I felt with the multitudes of tasks that the farm required nearly put me in an attorney's office. Brent was in love with the farm I often called "Lightening Hill." Stephanie loved it too. She is a lot like Brent in so many ways. She was a child in love with the dream her daddy was creating right before her eyes. He loved the barn work on the weekends. Scooping poop for hours gave him such great joy. Type As love organizing tasks and Brent was very good at this. He studied books and magazine articles on every animal we had and on every topic the farm could possibly encounter. It didn't keep the llamas from escaping at all hours of the day and night however. During arid seasons of the year the ground was too dry for the current to circulate through the soil and the fence, allowing the creatures to crawl through the wires.

Experiences create lessons books cannot prepare anyone for like accidentally leaving the barn door open allowing all 25 llamas to escape at once. I was talking to my girlfriend in the kitchen when one of the fuzzy creatures came up to the window looking for companionship. "Hummmm, have a treat in there for me?" Within seconds several more joined her. I laugh now but the panic, lack of organization and control almost put Brent over the edge! With friends visiting and the lack of accomplishing what he had expected Brent experienced more stress that day than he had a very long time. As for me, this had happened before. Stress and excitement were not going to resolve anything.

I work very well under stress. I don't like it, but I do it well. Often I wonder if this is one of the things Brent loves about me. I am willing to do things I don't like and do them well. He's even gone as far as to say "You don't know it yet but you'll like this." No, I probably won't like it but I'll do my best at it anyway. I, in my best Type B attitude, stayed calm and organized. I rounded up the ropes, the kids and a plan to get the escaped llamas back in the pasture. The llama escape day ended peacefully, and all was brought back to a sense of calm but the stress had worked its cruelty. Again, my peace and calm had been disrupted. I was angry and bitter about the way the situation had been handled and that I had to help out when the situation could have been resolved much differently. Brent was not accustomed to the escape artists yet. It would take a lot to rid me of my emotional state and I was not sure that would ever happen with my husband who I felt had little compassion for me in those situations.

Two years after moving onto the farm stress had worked its devastation on Brent too. His story of Fibromyalgia began here but I cannot blame it all on the experiences of the farm. Working 60 to 70 hours a week at this job, so far from his dream, and bringing some of that work home for evenings and weekends was affecting him as well. Stress, expectations and disappointment were creating the perfect condition for fibro to take control.

I had the pleasure of seeing authors Bill and Pam Farrel at a Hearts-at-Home conference several years ago. They wrote a book Men are Like Waffles, Women are Like Spaghetti. This analogy is so true for us! Brent gets into a project and stays there physically, mentally and emotionally for the duration of the project. I am a multitasker and I actually multitask my multitasks. I get into one project and then another, timing everything just right so I can come and go from one task to another and get everything accomplished at the same time. The intertwining of topics, tasks, and things together without losing sight of the original task is noodling or being like spaghetti. I am a "noodler." The "waffler" is most commonly described as a man who focuses on one task at a time and stays on task without disruption until the task is complete. Brent is most often a waffler and has a long list of projects to complete when the one he is doing is finished. Until I saw the presentation from the Farrel's I did not understand my frustration toward Brent about his lack of seeing a bigger picture. Many of our farm situations needed multiple tasks done at the same time, or accidents like gates being left open were going to happen.

Communication is huge in any relationship. Millions of couples go to counseling yearly to have a professional tell them what the other person is saying. Talking is very natural for most women. We often joked in our home that we girls had 25,000 words each, before feeling complete and finished at the end of the day. Brent felt he had 12,000 words to express himself on a typical day and he used them all at the office.[15] The lack of communication and the feeling that my needs and experiences during the day were not important began a break-down in our marriage and our every-day life. Where there is a break-down there is also possibility for rebuilding. I tell my girls, "Sometimes we need to fall apart so we can rebuild ourselves by rearranging all the pieces back together."

The farm offered multitudes of areas of growth for Brent and my relationship. There are no longer silent days in this house. They are simply not allowed. Conversations about conflict have at times taken on a more business-like manner. I write down what I see transpire in the issue of disagreement, how I feel it went wrong, and how I would try to alter my part of the responsibilities to help it change for the better. Fibro is also often questioned. Was he in pain and reacting or is this not related to fibro at all? I put a priority in getting my feelings out and verbalized. I do not however tell him how he should change. That is up to him. I also do not give more of myself to right the situation than I can give. Usually these conversations are one-sided. But, they do make a difference and change has happened.

The llama farm adventure lasted six years. I was ready for something else and Brent was ready for something more. God had a completely different direction for our family. Our next move was into a beautiful new home on two lovely grass acres. When we bought the 2 acres we were contracted to buy 35 more after selling the 18-acre farm. Brent had dreams of putting yak and zebu on the new farm with his llamas. Even the barn plans were all drawn up. The 18-acre farm sold and the transaction for the new 35 acres was ready for contract completion. The owner of the land had yet to have it surveyed, so we were told. As time passed so did the date of contract and the farmer decided not to sell the land to us. At the time we were crushed. Now, we see the good in the way the events played out. As the economy slowed, the land value decreased. We would have been in an upside down mortgage and very strapped for cash! If Brent had not been dealing with fibromyalgia and its struggles he would not have been open to seeing the other side of change. Sure, we would have had the dream farm, but I would have been miserable, Brent would have been driven to distraction and our marriage would have existed at best.

Now, we share more experiences happily together. The farm stress is gone. No more late-night escaping animals. No more sad deaths of new or old creatures on the farm.

I feel safe and peaceful; the girls have less distraction and disappointment. Now Brent can focus on what his passions are and take better care of his health. Much of the stress has been traded for quiet, peaceful times that bring us together.

Plans are good, organization has its place in chaos but we must not miss out on the small pleasures in life that make living enjoyable. We miss the smiles, little giggles, and glimmers of joy that are sprinkled throughout life when excessive demands are added to our lives. The plaster coat of pretty colors covers up the true creative side of life that resides below, and we lose sight of the foundational reason of why we are really here and that is to love and be loved.

On a Scale of 1 to 10

We are big ice cream fans. We love to try out new ice cream parlors and creameries. We even go as far as to take their flier and number their mixes and flavors on a scale of 1 to 4, with 1 being not great and 4 being awesome in flavor. We do this with simple decisions in life too. Do you like this paint color? Scale of 1 to 10? Do you want to go on a bike ride? Scale of 1 to 5? This brings us greater clarity in the decision-making process. Brent tends to be the kind of person who makes decisions at the 1 or 2 and 9 or 10 ends of the scale. He's more black and white in decision-making than me. I tend to sit on the decision and think about it.

There is a communication disconnect sometimes when I have not made a decision according to his process. I did not realize what could transpire if I didn't speak my thoughts about the question. To Brent it has been "we do this or we don't" and the decision is simply made right now. He does not think of whether this change or addition would create work or emotional stress. He believes we can let the solution play out and we will adjust. There is some validity to this thinking. I still have to watch my pauses though. The last time I paused too long he bought a cat.

One of the first things Brent told me after his Mayo diagnosis was that someone with fibro should not focus on the pain. He only evaluated the pain on his pain scale if it got excessive and stopped thinking of the pain any other time. How does one do that when they live with it daily? I thought if I knew his level of pain, maybe I could help make him feel better. It is a constant challenge for me to remember I am not responsible for his level of pain. I can do things that may help him feel more comfortable, like making healthy meals and snacks that benefit everyone in the family. Reducing excess noise in the house, scheduling family outings and activities in the mornings or afternoons also help eliminate heightened opportunity for fatigue. Leaving the evenings sacred for quiet time and preparing for bed have been great pain-reducing habits.

When Brent's pain started to exceed a 5 on a 1 to 10 scale I asked that he let me know. In knowing this I could prepare the girls to find quiet activities that would keep the noise level down. Noise and distractions are stimuli that enhance sensitivity in fibro sufferers. Too much noise can give Brent a headache. Too much stimuli like a family gathering can create too much activity and noise giving Brent fibro pain and extreme fatigue. He even gets exaggerated exhaustion if we go places with loud noises like a rodeo or with strobe lights at a concert. The television is just as much a culprit as the real thing. Depending on what activities he has participated in within the day, he can judge whether certain activities need to be altered or eliminated altogether for his best health and pain level.

There are ways to accommodate upcoming festivities, vacations or activities for the fibro sufferer. Physically slow down to rest and prepare for the upcoming event. Be one step ahead of the pain. If the event is going to be very busy, rest a little beforehand, and psychologically prepare the mind to eliminate the excess stress that may come. Give the body energy to cope with the added activity. Wearing ear plugs at a concert allows for musical pleasure but reduces the volume overload.

Communication breakdown with a person always in pain is so very easy to fall into. We don't want to be the reason for their pain. I tend to be very sensitive emotionally but I try to hide it well. Brent has no problem telling it like it is and finds humor in sarcasm as well. This confuses me completely. I sometimes don't know if he's frustrated, confused or serious. One time when visiting his brother they were bantering about snoring. I know this is the butt of many funny stories however this didn't seem funny when sleep in my house is so important. Brent often snores softly, but loud enough to keep me from returning to sleep, and as a light sleeper my sleep is crucial. In my sleeplessness I tried to gently roll his head to one side or the other to get the snoring to stop long enough to get back to sleep. Brent told his brother I "hit" him in his sleep. I took offence and corrected him only to have him repeat the scenario. They both understood the sarcasm and laughed. I became offended and left the room. I do not find sarcasm funny.

It is important to be sensitive to the level of activity and energy around us when fibro is involved but that doesn't mean we hide our feelings and not express them. I am a big advocate for always walking into a room by the way of the door. That way if I ever have to leave for any reason I know the way. I find it healthier to give visual, verbal, and physical space to situations that get unnecessarily elevated. This is helpful at the office, home, and family. Just a few minutes may be all that is needed to extinguish the heat of the moment. If it takes longer, you know where the door is. The time that it takes to cool down the situation may be the difference between serious pain and a simple inconvenience. Resolution may need to come later at a quiet moment, if at all. Although my feelings are acceptable and allowed, sometimes they are overly expressed and need time to calm.

It is so important for children to know their parent with fibro does not like being grouchy, but they need some quiet time to get grounded again. I am often heard saying "It is not your dad speaking, it's the fibro." Shortly after I explain this to the girls, I will wait for a quiet moment to tell Brent that he needs to remove himself from the situation (whatever it might be) before he loses it again. Usually he concludes that his pain was excessive and the situation could have ended much differently. The pattern is now set and when necessary, we have all learned to walk away from the situation before it gets out of control.

It is just as important for the child to feel they are heard. Programming the kids to be quiet due to disease can have lingering effects and create patterns that do not foster healthy communication. Often they need direction for their emotion and guidance for their feelings. We are the adults, fibro is the condition, and they need us to help them work through the challenges. Life is always a work in progress.

Our eldest, Stephanie, is a first born of two first born parents. She is one day going to be a great leader. She has many of Brent's leadership qualities. She is working on becoming more organized. As a teenager in the house she became challenging. She and Brent argued, often without resolution. He always wanted what was best for her. She wanted to find her own way through the situation. Both of their stubborn streaks got in the way. Separation, contemplation, and a little "mom intervention" helped bring them back together.

Extinguishing elevated problems need to be practiced by everyone. The girls and I would often go for a walk or pull out a quiet craft to help lessen the stress. Brent has taken up a few hobbies himself. His first real art hobby was beading. He beads beautiful small amulet bags. Here is where he escapes. He can relax completely. Even when his pain is escalating, he can calm himself in a quiet corner of the couch (no television or music usually) and bead. It is detailed and meticulous work but he loves it. It is fulfilling and peaceful for him. There is no stress involved. All the beading is done in his own time. He also quilts now. His beautiful throws are just as therapeutic as his beads and are just as fulfilling. Finding a relaxing, stress free activity for fibro sufferers is very beneficial. It allows the body to detach from life's stresses and enjoy a time away from the day-to-day activities.

Rainbow Hospice is our local non-profit hospice. It is new, beautiful, peaceful and loving. We do not plan on being patients there any time soon. Brent began volunteering as a patient visitor spending time with those that are in hospice and need a little companionship or supervision for a short period of time. He absolutely loves it! I see a future for him there.

Some people are not crafty or handy. There are many types of relaxation. Crafts are only one of the options for stress release. Feeling important and needed beyond the everyday life can help lower stress also. Volunteering at an animal shelter, hospital or hospice are very rewarding and refreshing, breaking the cycle of typical stress. These activities raise endorphins, make one feel good about what they are doing and ultimately lower stress and pain.

When one person in the family has fibro, everyone has fibro to some extent. It may not be physically, but environmentally and socially they do. By the end of the week we know Brent is affected by his fibro more severely. We try to steer clear of stressful situations and conversations. Timing is everything. For example if our youngest wanted to have a sleepover birthday party the topic should not be brought up on a Friday night. Having 10 teenage girls running around the house brings stressful thoughts to the father of this house. We time our conversations to happen when we feel they are best received. When this doesn't happen, and sometimes we have no control over our timing, like a fender bender, Brent has to find ways within himself to de-stress beyond his typical relaxation. Relief is not far away thankfully.

Every Saturday and Sunday night Brent takes a bath. Baths are also a great pain and stress reliever for him. It is believed that Epson Salt baths remove toxins in the body and help circulation.[16] Most fibro sufferers take a multitude of medications for their pain and sleeping. However, many may not be drinking enough water to eliminate the leftover toxins in the body. This is where the salts are said to help. He looks forward to Saturday and Sunday nights submerged in a hot bathtub of bubbles and a great book. He will be a new man when he reappears. On a scale of 1 to 10, a soak in the tub is a 10.

Healthy Fear

As a wife and mom, part of my job is helping to heal what ails someone. Kiss an "owie," wipe a tear, bandage a wound, and race to the emergency room with a broken collar bone are all in my job description. I live to help heal 24/7. Standing by a fibro sufferer is very difficult. I will support him in any doctor visits needed; although, it gets exceedingly frustrating when what appears to be a constant issue with a particular pain turns out to be unidentifiable.

My siblings and I often joked about injuries on the farm when we were growing up. If the injury wasn't severe enough to be life threatening or you were not turning blue or dying, then you didn't go to the doctor. Seeing a doctor has a different level of urgency now. "Back in the day" most people didn't have insurance and doctor's visits didn't cost several days' wages. Generations past went for issues that were beyond a day's rest, an at-home remedy, or a splint. That is not to say that all home remedies and rests created 'perfect' recuperation. I know elderly people with fancy looking scars and I have a finger that doesn't bend quite right. When going to the doctor didn't seem a priority, the visit didn't happen. In years gone by it was not about having a perfect body but a well-lived life.

A healthy fear can save your life. It can also cost a lot of time and money. Is it intuition, sixth sense or kismet? There are books full of mothers' intuitions. Stories are written of angels appearing out of nowhere. Where are the intuitions and sixth sense when my husband walks around holding his chest or stomach? He is always reassuring me it's just fibro pain. How do I know it's not a heart attack or appendicitis? I have to go on his word. I understand that fibro has a certain feel to the pain. I also know I have never experienced different "feels" to pain. Pain is pain. It all hurts and it indicates that something is wrong and needs attention.

Doctor visits happen much more freely today. I won't get into the politics of my belief why this is true, but I do believe that if we didn't have the opportunity to have insurance, and we were responsible for the cost of the visit, people would be making different decisions about their lifestyles and eating habits. Does this change conditions for the fibro sufferer? Probably not, but perhaps an evaluation would not involve so many separate professionals and at such great expense.

Unless Brent has a physical bodily injury or is not functioning normally, I let him decide his pain level and the need for professional care. However, if he's been injured, or acting out of character, then I step in. I think of it as having someone watching your back. At least I have better sleep knowing that his safety and health are not something I can control, but I can be there to support him. However, I have made a mental note of many an unusual groan or odd movement he has made in the past. I silently hold this information until I see it dissipate or discontinue altogether. If it doesn't disappear, then I approach the subject of his recent pain and health.

A few years ago Brent sporadically mentioned, "His ovary hurt." What ovary? With a laugh we went on with our day. Mentally I took a note. A month later he said it again. Several weeks later he said his right abdomen was achy. Ailments were beginning to add up. Life got busy with the girls starting school, work getting busy and life flew by for several months until Brent brought up his "ovary" again. He had already increased his pain vitamin and added a pain medication to help curb the severity of the discomfort. He thought perhaps his fibro was making the area feel worse than it actually was. No more mental notes. It was time to take action. After a visit to the doctor he found out that he had a hernia on his left and right sides of his lower abdomen. Surgery was necessary if he wanted relief from the constant pain.

For those of us without fibro, surgery is not something we want but know that if it is necessary we will do what it takes for ultimate health. It is different in sufferers of fibro. Medications react differently with fibro sufferers. Some work, some don't. Healing time is greater because they feel the pain of the surgery much longer than the rest of us.[17] Brent was skeptical but optimistic about the long range relief.

A few weeks prior to surgery he visited his general practitioner for a yearly blood draw for cholesterol. She put him on a different statin thinking it would be more effective. The old medication was actually working fine. She knew he had surgery in a few weeks and felt this change was fine.

His pain and symptoms continued up to and through the healing process. We thought his pain would be alleviated shortly after the surgery. Three days was normal and knowing Brent has fibro, we put that timeline out a little. The third day he had a fever, was shaking, had nausea, and was dizzy. His symptoms were getting worse not better. Within a week after surgery he lost the fever and shaking but he still had the nausea and lightheadedness as well as a lack of appetite. After a few weeks he went in to see if it was an infection that sometimes happens post-surgery. That came back negative. He continued to heal but the feeling of being in pain continued and because it felt intestinal or abdominal he thought it was hernia-related. Back to the surgeon for a follow up to eliminate whatever might be wrong. Again, they found everything to be healing normally. Even his general practitioner said the same thing after some blood work.

The pain and sickness and the lack of information was wearing on Brent. He was not denying that it could be fibro but would post-surgery discomfort really last for three months and really be this bad? A second opinion was necessary now. Actually, it was necessary a month prior. The new internal medicine doctor did a full check-up. He reviewed all his medication and noted all the symptoms. Apparently the new cholesterol medication was giving him negative side effects that mimicked post-surgery pain. The doctor put him back on his old statin and within two days he felt like a new person.

Without fibro, a person would have pursued the treatment very aggressively and doubted a doctor who found nothing. Having fibro, Brent often passed off the internal warnings that something was terribly wrong as just another side-effect of having fibro.

We all love answers to issues in life as long as they are helpful, useful and especially if they are positive. There are so many "advisors" in the world of pain. "Put ice on it, take vitamin such-and-such, see this doctor and try eating this diet." The list of advice goes on and on when dealing with a disease so vague in remedy. My advice is not to take on too many "advices." Take it slow. Get a good pain specialist and listen to your options. I am not a fan of medication; however, there are some out there that have been helpful to alleviate the pain. Be careful of the quick fix. There isn't one. Television advertisements are great forms of communication but they are not necessarily the answer. Their interest is to make money. Common sense plays a key role in pain control. Is it working? Are there unwanted or dangerous side effects that are worse than the fibro itself? Are there options that are more natural? A fibro person's health must not be overlooked just to alleviate pain.

We have looked at many such helpful options that claim to have few or no side effects. Brent was taking naproxen sometimes twice a day to take away most of the pain, but it was not improving his health, and he feared long-term side effects like an increased risk of heart attack or stroke, especially if you use it long-term or if you have a history of heart disease.[18] Naproxen may also cause stomach or intestinal bleeding, which can be fatal. These conditions can occur without warning while you are taking naproxen. With all the symptoms created by fibro, would anyone need this worry too?

There had to be better pain relief without the fear. I am not a doctor, nutritionist, or pharmacist. Going to the natural side of self-health is an unknown field to many and frightening for some. It takes some research too. If someone is not willing to put the time and energy into finding a safe alternative to pain relief then don't do it. Let a professional who has their own avenue of information do the work. That is fine and a good choice.

Brent started to look to natural remedies because I am a naturalist by heart. I go to the doctor if necessary, but I am a skeptic about the influence money and flashy studies have on the medical world. I'm not bashing it. I honor and have respect for all doctors and chemists. I just don't like what happens when money and advertising get involved. With that said, back to Brent. He started to go to a natural vitamin store in the area. The owner was very knowledgeable and a good sales person. They, too, desire to make a profit for a good living. Brent brought a small bottle of Curamin and a list of other products home to research before diving into the investment. The research had him asking questions to his health professional. What about his vitamin D level? Could there be a more natural way of lowering his cholesterol? Did he need the sleep aid? Everyone with or without fibro has the right to research their health if they chose to do so. Just keep it in perspective. Doctors have spent years studying and do want to help. Never make a major health adjustment without knowing if it is right for you from a professional vantage point.

The Curamin works wonderfully for Brent's fibro pain. The vitamin D increase has helped a great deal too. The vitamin for cholesterol did very little and the medication worked better. For several years he did not want to eliminate ice cream, cheese, and red meats from his diet. The increase in exercise and decrease in work hours was not happening either, so he continued the doctor's recommendation of medication.

Years later we have changed our eating habits. Being creative with healthy meals, I have slowly eliminated white flour and white sugar. Whole grains and other grains such as nut flours take white flour's place. Honey and maple syrup replace sugar. It is easy to substitute breads with fruits and vegetables to make the meals healthier. Today lasagna is a once a year treat and there's no ice cream in the freezer. There is less pain for Brent, while between the two of us many pounds have been shed. This worked for him. I like the healthy aspect. Brent has not completely eliminated his pharmaceuticals, although it is secretly my goal. He will however continue challenging pharmaceuticals and their health impact on his body.

Other forms of natural health remedies have also been researched by Brent. Magnets, essential oils, and prayer have all been a focus for him. Magnets had the fewest results scientifically, but he does wear a bracelet now and again claiming it improves his overall health. I do not get the same effect. I got a little dizzy when I wore it for an extended period of time and it made me uncomfortable.

The essential oils do have a lot more test results but come with a lot of usage instructions. Some oils can be ingested, some inhaled and others require topical application. Some oils can be used all three ways while others require a different combination. Brent likes the lavender as sleep aide and peppermint for muscle pain. He often comes to bed smelling very pleasant and whether I get a good night's sleep through osmosis or not, the room still smells nice!

Prayer and meditation has always been a part of our lives, but more so recently. A great deal of research has done in this area. The positive results are staggering; however, so is the skepticism. Does it work? Is it harmful? I am a believer. Is Brent pain free? No. But praying has its place enhancing patience and well-being and that is working.

Brent's father has had a minor stroke and his mother had a minor heart attack. These issues run in his family. Everyone has some sort of health history. What we do with this information is important. To be afraid of the future because of the "what ifs" in life creates undo stress that can bring about more illness. A person cannot go back and undo the past but they can at least learn from the past and alter the future.

A family with high cholesterol and heart disease needs to look at their diet and exercise. Are they eating enough fruits and vegetables? Perhaps their family genetics means they cannot digest red meats, fats or carbohydrates as well as another person. Drastically altering the diet early on may allow you to develop a system that does not pack fat on the body and cholesterol in the arteries. Perhaps exercise is lacking in a family. That too is a changeable behavior in one's life and can alter the way the body digests food and reduces stress.

A little history of Brent's family. They enjoy their meat, potato and bread dinners. For a portion of their lives both of his parents and even himself worked for a fast food chain. They took advantage of the convenient meals and ate there often. Back when they worked in these establishments I don't think the general public knew what they were eating; it was just convenient. Most fast foods don't contain sufficient dietary fiber and can lead to constipation. Studies are also finding fast food may cause a higher rate of depression. Convenient foods are high in refined carbohydrates, which can lead to fluctuations in blood sugar. If your blood sugar dips into hypoglycemic levels, you can experience anxiety, trembling, confusion and fatigue. With large portioned meals that are often high in fats, fast foods like burgers, fries and milkshakes deliver a hefty dose of calories as well. These large portions often leave you feeling full and lethargic.[19]

It is important to evaluate your family history too. Some families enjoy a good movie and several television programs on a daily basis. The amount of hours spent sitting is by far more critical than an exercise regimen they put into their regular lives. It may not be important to them. Could it change their overall health and happiness in life? Statistically, studies are showing exercise boosts brainpower and melts away stress. It strengthens your heart, lowers blood pressure, fights off disease, and increases your self-image.[20] There is always the question of how much is enough or too much. Most health clubs have trainers that can give exercise suggestions and if in doubt, get a check-up and ask the professionals.

Being focused on whether Brent will have heart disease or if he will suffer from a stroke is not emotionally or mentally healthy for me. Worry only creates stress. Eventually we will all die. My favorite quote is, "None of us makes it out alive." But I do focus on our comfort. If Brent were ever in extreme pain, we would be on our way to the emergency room. I cannot keep my husband living forever. We all will eventually go either by illness, old age, or the proverbial bus. If I can help make his life more pleasant by reducing stress at home, making healthy meals, and be a partner to make exercise more enjoyable, then my job as a wife and partner is complete, and my life is more enjoyable for me too. I might even indulge in a little mint chocolate chip ice cream from time to time.

In Sickness and In Health

Wouldn't life be wonderful if we knew that the "Happily ever after" was a guarantee in our lives? Those who believe in heaven know that there is no pain or suffering in eternity. Even that assurance sometimes doesn't make life any easier to live, with or without pain.

When my girls were one and three, before Brent had fibro, I began suffering from a headache. It came on in an instant and stayed for nearly 6 months. The severity of it fluctuated. Some days it was a nuisance, other days it was excruciating. There were days when I thought my head might split open. A true migraine raged for weeks at a time and medication barely helped. My doctor felt it was stress and gave me an antidepressant with some Advil. After several visits, he still felt no further action was necessary. I now know I should have questioned his diagnosis. A second opinion might have expedited the sense of urgency. Brent couldn't "fix" me either. He sometimes showed frustration toward me for not getting better. I couldn't just "buck-up" and shake it off.

If I look at all the variables involved I can see the picture much more clearly from today's vantage point. We were new parents with babies to care for. We had moved over a hundred miles from lifelong family and friends. Brent had begun a new job with more responsibilities than he had ever had before. We were taking on our first full makeover renovation. How many major life changes did that make? Brent's last straw was ready to break with me getting sick. He desperately wanted to put order into our lives but to no avail, and I couldn't help him. He reverted to his fight or flight mode. He fought to get me better by hoping he could will it upon me. His family relied on the doctor's say as final. The doctor said I had nothing wrong with me. Therefore, I should be able to shake it off and move on. The stress for me got greater and that increased his stress level too.

I have always had great health. The rare, few times I was sick I recovered in lightning speed. I have never suffered for long from much of anything. Even broken bones seemed to heal quickly, but, not this time. Brent really expected me to wake up one day and be healed. I honestly would have loved that too but it was not to be. I was blind to the severity of the symptoms. Pulling your head off the pillow by your hair in the mornings because it was too painful to lift should have been warning enough. But, it was not. For fun, our family went to a “Parade of Homes” one Saturday afternoon. I am an Interior architect by degree. I LOVE architecture! I should have been in my glory. Instead, I closed my eyes between rooms to eliminate excess stimuli and I sat on the curb between houses to rest to reduce some of the pain. Brent had no idea what to do. The doctor had the audacity to say I was fine.

After nearly six months, I suffered stroke-like symptoms. While getting the girls up from their naps I lost my speech and feeling in the left side of my face. I was terrified! With Brent an hour from home, I felt helpless. I feared I might die right in front of the children. Friends were called to take the girls, emergency personnel were called for assistance, and Brent was to arrive home shortly. The paramedics arrived and said all of my vitals were normal. There was no sign of any issue they could find that warranted me being taken to the hospital unless I chose to do so. All I had was confusion. I even fought the system to the last hour when the emergency paramedics told me that the ambulance ride to the hospital would be fifty dollars, if I was admitted. I sent them on without me to save the money. I knew I wasn’t leaving the hospital when I got in. What was going on? I was a healthy, active, young woman who was falling apart.

In the emergency room, the CAT scan results were not encouraging. I had what was called a subduralhymatomia. In common terms it was spontaneous brain bleeding between the brain and the skull. The brain surgeon was surprised to see I was still living. After a five-hour wait in the emergency room to gather the necessary personnel, I was prepped for surgery. The neurologist sat by my side the entire time, watching me and listening to my broken speech as I talked to Brent. At one point the surgeon took Brent out of the room and told him to go home and "prepare." The surgeon did not know if I was going to make it through surgery. Brent has said that has been one of the hardest and most stressful moments of his entire life. *I can only imagine*.

I have been on the side of pain that has no glory. I could not stop the pain. Brent could not take it away. I had no idea how to make life more livable. I also put my entire health in the knowledge of one man, the doctor. There is one factor I am leaving out - the largest part that kept me waking up every morning. That was my faith in God. I believed that although He didn't want me suffering, He did want me living. I was supposed to be a mother and wife through the pain. Learning how to execute even the simplest of my duties was challenging for everyone. The meals became simple, the house wasn't always clean and the perfection in our lives in general came to an aggressive halt. This may have confused and frustrated Brent too, but if it did, I was trying to survive and his desires for perfection would have to be altered at best. God had other plans. My existence became reliant on Him. No one else was going to get me out of bed to feed the girls. The medication didn't touch the pain, the doctor wasn't fixing anything, and Brent was at a new job in a start-up situation; he couldn't be home to help. This was the time in my life when faith was challenged, and it only brought me to a greater sense that this life is only temporary. In the big picture of eternity, human life was a drop in the bucket and this temporary period of pain even less so.

Obviously I survived. I even woke up the next morning to see the doctor who had misdiagnosed me for months kneeling at the foot of my bed. It was a true miracle that I came through so well. Do prayers work? I know there were hundreds, if not thousands, of people with me in their prayers that night. I am going to thank them all by saying, "Yes, all of the prayers worked!" After the successful surgery I regained strength quickly and resumed my healthy lifestyle within six months. The surgeon complimented my progress. I have had no other reoccurring issues since. My rally for life is stronger than it has ever been and I will do all that I can to remain healthy, because those six months were the hardest lessons I have ever learned and the most life experience education I will ever need.

After spending many years being afraid of having another bout of brain bleeding, I spent some time evaluating what I had been going through in my life that may have contributed to that condition. If I could change the behaviors that surrounded the situation, perhaps I could reduce the chance of it happening again. Stress was an overwhelming factor in my life at the time. I think I knew it was a problem but I had no idea how to confront it or reduce it. There was a slow fade from living a quiet life before having children to the crazy and chaotic life that came after moving to Wisconsin. Increasing responsibilities automatically happen when children are added to a family, but the home renovation caused me to feel like I was careening out of control. I felt that I had no voice. After all, I was not bringing any financial contribution into the household any longer so what right did I have to complain? I don't think Brent had any idea of my distress either. He was so wrapped up in the responsibilities of his new job, he didn't have the energy to see what was happening to me.

I do remember a time before surgery, when the girls were watching television and I was making lunch for us in the kitchen. The pain in my head was so tremendous that I sank to the floor and asked God to help me survive. The tears flowed silently as I released my overwhelming feelings of helplessness to God. I had what I call a blessing at that moment. I felt the presence of God with me and knew I was being cared for and loved. God did not care if I was painting the house to make it beautiful or stripping varnish to remove unwanted grime. God wanted me just as I was. He saw me and loved me without expectations. That moment lasted long enough to allow me to continue on with life but it didn't change my behaviors.

The path of life looks much different when we turn around and look back. I see that without my brain surgery I would not have my tremendous love and respect for my relationship with God. This helped change my behaviors and habits. Almost losing my life made me look at my purpose here in a different way. I am not supposed to be a worker-bee without consideration for myself. I am looking out for my well-being now and relishing the opportunity to help others see their self-worth as well. The gift of my experience has been the ability to relate to others who are in pain or have tremendous confusion about their life. I feel a connectedness to them and their search for inner peace. Perhaps I had to learn this prior to Brent's fibromyalgia so I could have understanding and compassion toward him in his times of pain and confusion. I also think I was blessed with this experience to know how to care for myself in times of great stress. I need to put my health first, before I can help others be healthy.

It has taken many years to grow into the person I have become today, and I am ever changing. One of the hardest things to remember, as a spouse of a fibro sufferer, is that I do not cause the pain nor can I take it away. "For better or for worse" are words practiced on a regular basis in our marriage. I often feel when Brent is in a lot of pain that he looks to me to do something to make it better. Part of my being the "nurturer," I guess. I know I am not to blame, but even more so, I need to separate myself from the responsibility of taking away his pain.

In Good Times and In Bad

Work hard, play hard, live harder. Brent moves through life at break-neck speed sometimes. When I can't, or won't, keep up with his desires, he sometimes becomes frustrated. Trying not to take it personally is not easy, but I know that at times I need to be the voice that brings life to a slower pace.

He is gradually getting the point that life was meant to be enjoyed, even savored, and not conquered. He has told the girls, "It is not the product but the process that is to be enjoyed." I know he says it, now to put it into action. Perhaps his pain is starting to show him how to slow down and enjoy the process as well. Life is a masterpiece of growth and adjustments; some are painful and some are pleasurable but all are part of the process.

Encouraging healthy eating, early bedtimes, simple exercise, quieting excess noise, offering help for a creative outlet like quilting are all part of my "wifely" role now. There are times when our lives fall into a hurried rush. Prior to fibro, this was a normal lifestyle. I was often heard saying our vacations were very much like Clark Griswold's, the character played by Chevy Chase. We have actually visited several large attractions in one day. We have visited a Wildlife Park, SeaWorld, and a Deer Park all on the same day while driving out to visit relatives in New York. We had never done anything spontaneous before. Everything had a plan. This trip however started out as a day trip and ended up being a long four-day weekend. Our one-year-old had few complaints, but as a new mom I was ready to jump ship. Trying to entertain, feed, and bed an infant without a packed suitcase almost put me over the edge. We did find a superstore and purchased what we needed, and the spontaneity of the trip was exciting, but those trips have been few and far between. I respect the need to get away but not at neck-break speed. It has taken years to slow him down but I believe he is learning. The alarm clock is not set during vacations and we visit only one main attraction a day. Control is one thing but out-of-control creates too much stress and lack of enjoyment.

Our second child has been attributed to slowing us down in the early years. Alexis is our "Stop and smell the roses" child. When we were in a rush she was finding just the right shoes, searching for the perfect perfume and enjoying the process. There have been times when I felt that if I could just slow down the moment, I might catch something I'm missing. We rushed from riding lessons, to a game and then off to a birthday party hours away. Craziness! As the "other half," I know now that part of my responsibility is also to put on the brakes. I know I can't make Brent stay home from his activities. I do know that if I don't want to go because I need to slow down, perhaps he may choose to do so also. If he doesn't, well, that's his choice. I have a rule, actually two rules. All plans must be made at least 24 hours prior to the event, and we only do one thing or go one place each weekend. Everyone gets the ability to be spontaneous without chaos and I get a quiet afternoon at home at least once a week. Brent sees the slower life as better and is actually more enjoyable. However, his responsibility to his work and his desire to have a slower life are in conflict each other. We do have fewer agendas for the weekends and every now and then he enjoys a weekend with little to do. Having a stressful schedule is unhealthy. I cannot make him see this though. He must see it for himself. Otherwise, he is changing for me and not himself and that is not a stress-free lifestyle either. It is all part of personal growth and I respect that.

The girls also needed to see an active healthy lifestyle. They enjoyed going to all of their activities but there needed to be a limit. When we parents can set healthy limits to our activities while they are young, then they will be able to set healthy limits for themselves in the future. One of the girls might have asked to go to a friend's game or out shopping at the last minute. We do not live near town. If these plans were made only a day before, then transportation and meals could have been arranged. We have a friend who encourages their children to go out for several sports at one time. Granted that's admirable to allow them such choices. But to be involved in swimming and volleyball at one time, or track and softball and to have more than one child in different sports would be complete chaos for me! I actually did not get a lot of complaining about activities missed. I think the girls enjoyed the down time as much as the active times, as long as they were evenly balanced.

Our family loves vacationing in tourist areas. We have a process that actually works. Brent finds activities in the area and the rest of us try to pick the top item of the day that we would all like to visit. No more Clark Griswold planning on our trips. The greatest part of the trip however is in entering the hotel and finding the room and its accommodations. We love the mystery of it. We are not campers. A room with a shower, television, and two beds is not too much to ask for but we do have our limits. Then, as usual, we rate it at the end of our stay on a 1 to 4 scale. Would we return? There have actually been hotels that were supposed to be a multiple nights' stay and we checked out after one nights' stay due to poor accommodations. There are other hotels that we have extended our stay for extra nights. Spontaneity and organization all in one vacation, perfect.

Being a spouse to a person with fibro is not as easy as just "checking out!" I know there are days when tempers flare and the option to bale seems easy, after all the lifestyle is not as we once hoped. We married into the relationship for better or for worse. There are going to be times when the accommodations or communications are going to have to change. Keeping peaceful communication is tremendously important, difficult but important. Angry words, bitter looks, distasteful undertones only cause greater stress and poorer communication in an already challenged situation. Chronic pain and debilitating fatigue are not like a tattoo. The sufferer did not ask to have fibro; they would like their physical life the way it was before. We did not expect fibro to be a part of our lives either. We together must deal with it lovingly, openly, and as peacefully as possible. This is not to say that being dumped on and treated poorly is acceptable by any means. All parties involved must participate in open, honest, and peaceful communication. Raising voices, stomping around, and keeping up a silent front are stress builders, destructive to relationships, and increase pain.

We may never see a cure in our lifetime for fibro however, I know that in reducing stress and continuing to support my husband through peaceful communication, healthy eating and some spiritual prayer, we will all live a much happier life.

Who knows? Maybe a stress-free life is the cure. No drugs, no needles, no doctors, just stress-free living as a cure. Now wouldn't that be heavenly?

Reality Check

When Brent and I were first dating, he was from the "city" and I was a "country girl." Prior to being married he said that he was going to one day own llamas. I laughed. I was graduating from college in interior architecture and was not planning on returning to the country. Plans change, life is altered and, yes, we bought the farm.

When we lived on the farm I loved the gardens, the yard, and the scenery. I did not love the animal escapes, the vet visits and the seventy-hour work weeks Brent spent away from home. Brent loved caring for and cleaning up after the animals. It was far from euphoric but there were parts that we truly enjoyed. We owned 25 llamas, 6 pigs, 50 chickens, 10 cats, 3 sheep, and a dog at the height of living on the farm.

There was joy in raising the animals and gardens. It was a little slice of heaven. Beauty was everywhere. Although when Brent began showing signs of fibro, life came to a quick halt. We honestly thought he had something terminal. Seventy hours of work a week is enough stress for a person, let alone keeping up a farm. Brent would have loved to quit his job and farm for a living but we needed his paycheck to pay the mortgage. After struggling with the fibro and the farm for two more years, we decided to sell the current farm and buy new. It was one of the hardest decisions we have ever made but one of the wisest. We now have lots of time for the girls, ourselves and our remaining pets.

Laughter is the best medicine.[21] There are few remedies for difficult times that have such a positive impact. We are slowly incorporating this value into our family lifestyle. Brent and I had rather serious careers before I became a full-time mom. Now only he has the serious career. Alexis again helps bring perspective to a situation. Try as we might we cannot force her to pick up the pace or change her inner self. With Alexis, there always seems to be a silver lining and a positive side. Stephanie likes to procrastinate. This drives us all crazy but there is a lesson to be learned. Although what needs to be done is important, so is living and sometimes the priorities need to be altered to get in a little more living. Because of their outlooks the girls are full of creative joy. They are continuously reminding me that life is not to be taken so seriously.

We have an open -concept kitchen, dining room, and living room. I spend the majority of my time in the kitchen. I love the kitchen. The girls are true girls; they giggle all the time. They are often teasing each other about something and laughing. When their friends are over they become entwined in the silliness and the giggles continue. I wouldn't trade overhearing this for anything. Recently, I realized I needed more of this in my life. I enjoyed hearing it, why not engage in it? Fibro is serious. I needed to lighten up in order to enjoy more time with my family.

Every night the family sits down together for dinner and shares their daily events. Brent sometimes brings interesting news clippings home for conversation. We try diligently to keep supper a family time. There have been times where supper is at 8:00 p.m. due to practice of some sort but we share supper together.

I am an open and honest person. If it needs to be said, I say it. My openness has created quite a lot of laughter around the table, especially when the friends are over. Conversations get real. Boyfriend silliness, the reality of humanness, and questions to encourage growth are all part of a healthy meal conversation at our house. My girls often roll their eyes with an, "Oh mom…" as everyone laughs.

Fridays have always been pizza night. I love homemade pizza. It gives me great joy in making it and in eating it. The meal is simple and the set-up and clean-up are easy. The conversation, however, is challenging by Friday night. Brent has given 110 percent all week at work and by Friday night he's had it. He's exhausted. A year after diagnosis we figured out the system. When talking to Brent at the dinner table on Fridays, one must wait for him to acknowledge you, look at you, and then listen to you. All three of these must happen or he's not with you. We laugh now. He's often in his fibro fog[22] while we talk. I know he says we are always talking. We're girls. But, his fibro fog has brought us all endless joy. Laughter abounds when he sits glazed like a doughnut and about as responsive.

One of the side effects of fibro is fibro fog. We now refer to Fridays as Fibro Fridays. On Fridays we do not ask Brent to do any major decision-making, take on large projects or travel long distances. The mind goes into neutral and idles there. No response. This can be dangerous when driving or using large tools. Neither of which we ask Brent to do on Friday evenings. Fibro Fridays are also full of dropping things. Brent can't hold an object without dropping it by Friday night. Ladies in his office laugh about this too. Papers, pencils and books all greet the floor eventually on Friday if Brent is holding them.

We are not making fun of Brent but making light of a situation that could be very frustrating for him. We do not try to make him feel foolish, only loved for who he is during his difficult times. There is little to be done to correct Fibro Fog or Fibro Fridays. Laughter is the best medicine. This happens when we help him reconnect to the conversation by giving him a pleasant reminder such as what it was our oldest was talking about when he zoned out or picking up the forks when they hit the floor. It is all done with love and makes it so much easier to laugh about.

The disease of Fibromyalgia is no laughing matter. More and more people are diagnosed with it every year. Doctors find no pre-diagnosing patterns in their patients. Every symptom is different and can be of different severity per individual. With no true pattern of preventative treatment or cure, most doctors are stymied in where to start. One thing is a constant for all sufferers: stress. Stress is a huge factor in the amount of pain a person with fibro feels. The greater the stress, the greater the pain one feels with fibro. Even times of great joy can be very painful. My girlfriend, who suffers with fibro pain, was overjoyed when she learned of her son's engagement. An engagement, is a very joyous time but planning a wedding and watching your child leave home is very stressful. Extra quiet time and extra self-care are a big help in reducing pain. As a spouse, sometimes helping to see unnecessary activities or participation as a detriment to staying out of pain is difficult but beneficial in the overall enjoyment of the festivities.

Weather also has a great deal to do with pain. During the months of November, December, January, and February, Brent is in heightened state of pain. Cold rain, snow, bitter temperatures and any mix of these are horrid for fibro sufferers.[23] We have often thought of moving to a warmer climate. So far we are still in Wisconsin, but the weather is not going to keep us here, that is for sure. I do keep the temperature of the house up a little higher than I want, for Brent's comfort when he's home. When we vacation, we go to warmer and dryer climates like Colorado and Arizona. Our time is spent relaxing, sightseeing, hiking and de-stressing. Brent's pain is almost nonexistent when we are in these areas for vacation.

We dream of our future often. Now that we are "Empty nesters" what will we do? Where will we go? I think if we didn't have fibro in our lives we'd be looking at different options. We are looking at relocating to that "pain-free zone" for retirement. We keep asking ourselves if we need to wait that long. Can we wait that long? Will fibro wait for that time? What is his window of pain tolerance? And of course that proverbial bus is always looming. At what point does one say enough working the daily grind to make a mortgage payment and chose to live instead. Of course there are the few people I read about who are doing both, but reality is most of us are working to pay for a mortgage and a vacation every now and then, with dreams of one day living differently. The American dream of a large house, 2.5 kids and a pet have disappointed most of us, and the new dream is to love what you do and foremost do what you love. Now, what is that exactly?

Fibro in the Work Place

One of Brent's greatest fears is missing work or eventually not being able to work at all.[24] According to government statistics, only 15 to 20 percent of fibromyalgia sufferers are currently on long-term disability.[25] It has only been since 2012 that Fibromyalgia has even been considered severe enough to be a disability.

In the past few years there have been governmental guidelines drawn up for the employer to help keep conditions in the workplace more pleasant for people diagnosed with fibromyalgia. The lists can be obtained at https://askjan.org/media/Fibro.html. The U.S. Department of Labor's Job Accommodation Network list contains recommendations for accommodations employers should be willing to consider for employees with fibromyalgia.

Employers should consider the following:

- Providing written job instructions when possible
- Prioritizing job assignments and providing more structure
- Allowing flexible work hours and allowing a self-paced workload
- Allowing periodic rest periods to reorient
- Providing memory aids, such as schedulers or organizers
- Minimizing distractions
- Reducing job stress [26]

There are a few items on this list that Brent does not and probably feels he cannot follow. He has a busy job overseeing human resources, marketing, insurance, office administration and so much more! The stress level at this job for him is crazy. Although his Day-Timer has it all planned out it is still unbelievable. He has often said he has meetings every quarter-hour or the day is full from the moment he gets in. This includes the days he is traveling. He will pack the airport wait time with a conference call or answering emails. We have even experienced him interviewing a candidate for the office while on a vacation away from home. His stress level at the office is off the charts as far as the U.S. Department of Labor goes. He feels there isn't time for quiet breaks or a flexible schedule when he has so many people relying on him to keep things running smoothly. Step into his office and the definition of business takes on a different look in the work place. There is great fear in today's world of losing your job because of failure to perform what is required even if it means sacrificing one's health.

Looking at the list above, Brent has executed what he can with diligence and purposeful attention. He goes in earlier than most employees to get a head-start on work while it is quiet. This is a sacrifice to his sleep but a help to his work. He also lives, and I do mean live, out of his Day-Timer. The Day-Timer is his heart beat at work. He writes EVERYTHING in it. Without it he is lost. Brent keeps every phone conversation, meeting, message, and schedule of events in his Day-Timer. I even show up in there now and then if I have to call him about something. His organizational skills are off the charts! He has got this part of his life under a written form of control.

The list above requires a work environment with minimal distractions. Many people work in cubicles or less. These small spaces with half partitioned walls do not allow much privacy or keep-out distractions. People walking by, noises from conversations just down the way, or phone calls can be very distracting. Brent has a door on his office that cuts down on disruptions and noise, which helps quiet his environment, although employees can knock or make an appointment if they need to talk to him. As long as he has the time, he will see whoever needs him.

An additional aid to his treatment of fibro is his attention to his nutrition. He eats breakfast in his car on the way to work. Usually breakfast consists of a piece of fruit or yogurt. Before being diagnosed, he skipped breakfast because he doesn't like breakfast foods. He has found without breakfast he quickly loses energy and patience and is starving by lunch. Lunch is usually a left-over from supper the night before or a frozen left-over from a previous meal. These lunches are quick, nutritious, and healthy. They are not full of preservatives, fats, salts, or sugars that can slow a body down after being eaten. He doesn't give himself a lot of time to eat and usually he is at his keyboard while eating so these meals are perfect. On his way home he will indulge in a snack, but again, it is healthy like nuts and dried fruits.

At the office my husband is famous for his notes. His notes are at home too and they help him feel organized. I'm not fond of them and I find little pleasure in them. His assistants however, find his notes helpful, articulate, sometimes a little annoying, and even humorous. The purpose is to eliminate confusion and excess stress at the office and it does work. I've even heard him referred to as "Mr. Post-it." He knows his message is relayed, physically, and the employees know what he needs and when. This is a great form of organization for Brent and helps him feel in control of the little pieces of his work place.

Every Saturday he makes and executes his notes at the house. He even adds things like "call dad" or "bathe the dog" on these notes. They appear silly to me so I have no notes. Why should I make notes when he has so much on his list needing my assistance that mine will never see daylight or appear important? I will admit there are times I frustrate myself by forgetting something. I do force myself to write a grocery list although Brent has usually started it before me. Every once in a while I will make a phone call list but that's it. It is a personal issue I suppose. I go to the opposite extreme of Brent. He makes lists of everything therefore I make none at all.

Brent is someone who gives 110 percent. I don't think he'll ever really retire. He will just move from one profession to another with maybe a few less demands. He likes to work. He likes the fulfillment of the challenge, the accomplishment of successfully executing a difficult concept. He's quoted as saying "Give me a problem and I'll find an avenue for the answer in 3 phone calls or 3 web surfs." I believe he can do it too!

The Easy Button

I love the television advertisements with the "Easy Button." This advertisement has me thinking of so many possibilities. What's for dinner? Easy Button…done. What choice of clothes for my picky dresser? Easy Button…done. Is Brent in pain? Easy Button…GONE.

Sadly, there is no easy button for living. There is however growth. We are all on this earth on our own journey. We are not alone but individually on separate journeys. I can no more make your life end perfectly than you can alter mine for the same reason. We can, however, be there for each other and lend a hand when necessary. We can be the listening ear, the helping hand, the shoulder to catch a tear. It is not easy taking care of others, though, if we are not taking care of ourselves.

We are barraged with infomercials about exercise machines, diet pills, eating plans and other details of living that we are supposedly lacking. One very important factor to remember about all of these advertisers is that even though they mean well they are out to make money. A smart start to self-health care is having a healthy image. You may be overweight, short, balding, wrinkly, or a combination of other negative self-images that plague you, but remember you are loved by others and worth every breath you take. Regardless of your external looks and fears of what others might think of you, you alone are the only wonderful you. There are people who look for you when they walk by your house. Someone is silently smiling because of something you said in the past that made them feel good. You are a part of someone's memories and thoughts. In knowing this alone, everyone is wanted and needs to take care of oneself.

Emotionally, it is difficult to be a continuous supporter of someone in pain. Life does have its pains. We are survivors. We are needed. We are loved. One minute life deems to fly by and we are heard saying, "Where did the time go?" And another day when we are being challenged we feel like time could not crawl any slower. Each day will have its challenges to conquer. Some we will feel were successful, others we will perceive as failures. There is nothing we do that does not have a purpose. I once had a girlfriend ask, "Who is your cheerleader?" Good question. There are days I feel like I am on a journey unlike any other without much appreciation. I do know the appreciation is there, just sometimes not expressed. We caregivers are appreciated. What we do is seen and commendable. Often we don't hear that enough but we are. Perhaps it is all in our perception.

For some of us, getting motivated to keep ourselves physically healthy can be underwhelming. Going alone for a walk or bike ride can seem boring. Taking those who love us along on our healthy journey makes it a lot more fun and gets them up and moving as well. A fibro sufferer needs exercise to help keep their body working healthfully and efficiently. Research has shown a large improvement in pain management when the fibro sufferer exercises on a regular basis.

Exercise can be intimidating. While in college I lifted weights, did aerobics and walked a lot. I was healthy and fit. While pregnant, I took swimming exercise classes for expectant moms. After childbirth I enrolled in aerobic and step-fitness classes. Today, on a few acres, in small town America, there are few places that offer any type of fitness within a 15 mile drive from the house. To get motivated to workout when I have to get into the car and drive a measurable distance is not encouraging for me. I realize that for college, pregnancy and post-baby I had a friend join me in the workout. The travel time and self-talk was not a deterrent to a good workout when I had a friend meeting me there. Moving to the country was beautiful, but beauty does not come with an exercise routine. I used to think the farm work was enough of a work out for a healthy body. I was just kidding myself. It is true that keeping up with a large yard and small farm are a lot of work. It is not well-rounded enough to make it a good and complete workout. Plus, seldom do I find a friend who will come over to help pull weeds or rake grass. Asking Brent to help is a stretch but if I can offer to help him, he usually will offer to help me and we enjoy the work required to keep the yard looking nice. We both win physically and have fun at the same time.

I do not think I look good in biker's shorts, but that doesn't stop us from heading out when the weather is conducive to a peaceful and stress-free bike ride. We don't go far but we get out in the fresh air and enjoy each other while exercising. On a bike path nearby, there is a beautiful little bridge that covers a stream full of frogs and small fish that has become our resting place. We try to make the trip as enjoyable as possible. To exercise you don't need a gym or a track. A simple walk around the neighborhood or the local shopping mall is good enough. The most important factor is to have a friend along. That also goes for the fibro sufferer as well. As with any exercise program, your doctor will know what is best for you if there are physical conditions to be considered.

Our rides have encouraged Brent's competitive edge as well. Thankfully it is not against each other but against a personal best. He takes count of the number of miles and calculates them at the end of the summer. He hopes to surpass the previous years' mileage by the end of the season. We also like to challenge ourselves by riding on the road. The bike path is nice, tree covered, car free, and flat. The road is none of these. By the end of the season we will ride into town and back again. He feels a great sense of accomplishment.

Many studies have been done on exercise and stress. A regular exercise program can slow down the heart-racing adrenaline associated with stress, but it also boosts levels of natural endorphins that are pain-fighting molecules. Endorphins help to reduce anxiety, stress and depression.[27] Make exercise fun, relaxing and enjoyable. Make the things you like doing a form of exercise. A visit to the zoo, art museum or walking the dog in a park are all good starts to a creative exercise program. Make it fun, make it often, and include your friends. With habits like these you are on your way to a much healthier lifestyle.

Identifying favorite exercise activities needs to be right up there with identifying stress areas in our lives. If it creates stress it needs to be stopped or at least altered. There is no physical advantage in having stress in one's life. There are countless ailments that are attributed to stress: heart attack, ulcer, migraine, back pain, to name a few.

Too often we make up excuses for the stress. "I've always done it this way." "There is no one else who can do it." "I have a schedule to meet." Really? All these statements are close-ended minded decisions. Be creative. Make small alterations at first. Put some time between you and the request. If you do not take care of you, no one else will. Those with fibro are constantly challenged with their pain. We are often challenged to fit our needs and desires into their schedule. We fibro caregivers need to take on as much of a stress-free life as possible. It is time to make small changes and keep going. These will slowly accumulate into more stress-free activities, creating a stress-free life for everyone.

I have often heard that being a mirror to someone will eventually reflect back nicely. Be a mirror of limited stress. Show how to arrange life stress-free. When you find yourself in an unusual or stressful decision, alter the difficult activities and make them enjoyable. Perhaps in time, life will begin to reflect back through the fibro sufferer and be a much less stressful lifestyle.

We are here for the long haul. There are times when maintaining a loving and healthy relationship is very difficult. I know that being pushed to the edge of frustration is not desirable, but, neither is having fibro. This is another challenge, an obstacle to get around. Again, there are no "Easy Buttons," only understanding that you are not alone. An unsettled relationship holds a lot of stress and sadness, none of which helps a fibro sufferer or their spouse. If necessary, take the first step to a healthier relationship and contact a professional. Living with limited stress and a healthy exercise program will create a joy-filled lifestyle without dreaming of the "Easy button."

Valid Questions

So, you know your spouse or significant other has Fibromyalgia. You've heard the doctor's diagnosis and options. What about you? Is there treatment for the "other half?" As of today the "family and friend" factor of fibromyalgia has very limited support. We are a silent group hurting on the inside but saying very little. There are few support groups for us. I suggest that you find an outlet for fun, a friend you trust, and a group you can relax with. We helpers often throw ourselves into the servant mode and forget to care for ourselves. Finding a group of friends who are happy, healthy (mentally), and supportive is a very good way to take care of yourself.

Will your spouse get worse? No crystal ball here. No one knows. However, I can tell you that there are many ways to improve your way of living and help you enjoy life a little more. I have heard it takes seven repetitions to make a habit and 21 times to break it. We are developing habits to create comfort all the time even discomfort is a comfort for some. I have heard "At least you know the devil you are working with." That may be so but it could be destructive to your health. It will take time and perseverance to re-train the habit into something positive. Exercise, eating, sleeping and stimuli are all alterable. Get creative, have fun, and make an effort that will make a difference.

My youngest went to a civil war reenactment with her school and brought home some fun and interesting facts. There is one story that is used often in humor around here. She was told that in a particular Indian tribe the wife could put her husband's moccasins outside the teepee door if she wanted him to sleep outside or, more drastically, wanted a divorce. Today we joke when Brent gets himself in the doghouse that I am going to put his moccasins out on the porch. It brings humor to a situation that is getting out of hand and is uncomfortable to confront. One still confronts the situation but more gently and in a manner that the girls can learn from and I can deal with. I do not enjoy confrontation but I become stressed if I don't deal with the issue in a quick and timely manner. The issues tend to "stew" if I postpone them and get more intense. I ruminate on the issue and I over-analyze what may be causing me stress. This just creates more stress and is usually not accurate. Then, when other issues accumulate, I just get angrier until I lose it. That is never a good thing. To break this habit I need to stay focused on the issue at hand. If the situation cannot be resolved in the instant, then I need to resolve to work on the issue later. I try not to allow myself to rehash the situation over and over in my head. It will be there to think about later, and if I forget about it later or perhaps for a very long time, then maybe it wasn't that big of a deal to begin with. Time may put some perspective to the entire situation and allow it to dissipate all on its own.

Some days are diamonds, some days are stone. When will the happy days return? Yes, there will be hard days. Yes, there will be days you will never want to end! Only now, you may have to look a little harder for the gem-like moments in those days. Keeping a positive outlook is very important for both of you and especially if you have children! They are watching you. They are learning, silently from your actions and communication. Fibro is not going away. The likelihood that your children will know someone else in their life with fibro is very probable. What will they take with them into their relationships in the future? Work on showing them less stress, better eating habits and the importance of sleep. Expressing healthy communication, allowing some time out for contemplation, and seeking resolution with a healthy dose of unconditional love are all tools will last a good long lifetime.

What about the big "D?" A shocking 75 percent of marriages with a fibro-suffering spouse end in divorce according to statistics!![28] The odds are stacked against us![29] I can tell you that Brent and I have passed by that thought a few times. We have used it in anger. We have used it in passing. We DON'T use it any more. Divorce is a defeatist, fighting word. It is an unfair way to fight if used in anger. Fibro is not an affair; it is not abuse. Fibro can create situations that feel unfair or possibly abusive and in these situations professional help is advised.

Be a supportive spouse is some advice I can give. I didn't say touting, sacrificing, or suffering spouse. We must stay true to our journey and encourage our loved ones along the way. It is my observation that the fibro sufferer keeps their pain sheltered within their daily routine. My friends with fibro say that unless you look ill or have reason for pain people do not understand the pain. Therefore they believe others do not see them in pain. This is true and must be very frustrating for the fibro sufferer. As you know, the sufferer often endures the pain privately and alone. They no more want sympathy from others than you do. But some compassion, understanding, and perhaps a listening ear is a good start.

I believe we are all on an independent journey on this earth together. We each have a desire or passion that drives our lives. Fibromyalgia is part of the sufferer's journey, not ours. Remember, we can no more change their life's journey as they can change ours.

With compassion for the sufferer, I must discuss a serious side effect of fibromyalgia: Depression. How serious is this depression? Suicide takes about 10 percent of women who have this painful disorder.[30] If you suspect your spouse is nearing a destructive pattern of behavior, it is time to take action. Don't wait and see! There are many professionals out there that specialize in severe depression. Your spouse is not choosing to be in pain. They are possibly choosing a destructive way to deal with it. They are not "nuts," or "insane." They are in pain and need additional help that is not available at home. You are not to blame for not offering the right support, love, or encouragement. They simply need more than what you can provide.[31] This is okay! It is good to encourage help. You have addressed the depression straight on. It is also good to go with them and be there to support them as they get help. You, too, are going to need a little support.

"Just keep swimming, just keep swimming," Dory in Disney's movie *Finding Nemo* said it well. Will I ever be able to do enough? We are human beings but we really should be called "human doings." No, you will never be able to cure fibro. You cannot take it away no matter what you do, say, invent or discover. If you do, you'll be one wealthy person! So, just be there, support, listen, help and love the person you know who has fibro. They don't want to be loved any less than if they didn't have fibro.

Finding the delineation line between you and them is so important. Where do I begin and the fibro end? As a caregiver it is easy to be blended into the situation. Like smearing the line, we give a little more than comfortable and they take what is offered. Fibro is new to us all. There are no two patients alike. There are no two relationships alike. But, there are two distinct people in your marriage, one with fibro and one without. It is ok to take care of you and them. Taking time out for yourself to rejuvenate and reconnect with who you are is important to you and your spouse! They fell in love with you and they don't want to lose that person to the fibro. Staying on your journey keeps you strong and helps them too.

It's the differences that make the difference. Will I get Fibromyalgia too? First and most importantly, fibro is not contagious, viral, or bacterial. You will most likely never get fibro because you are different from your spouse. You do not have the same emotional system. You resolve conflict differently, deal with stress differently, and live life differently. Is your lifestyle better? Not necessarily, just different and not fibro enhanced. We do, however, need to keep that system grounded and at peace. Spending some time in peace and quiet is a great way to stay emotionally and physically healthy. Our decision-making skills are sharper and our stress level is lower. We can act more efficiently in stressful situations and make better decisions in challenging conditions when we give ourselves regular, quiet down time.

We want to make plans for the future. What can I expect? Well, there will always be plans made, plans changed and spontaneous plans. In a family living with fibro, plans need to be flexible but definite. There are times Brent wants to stay home due to exhaustion and pain. There are also times we go and take the day at half speed. Sit on a bench and let the girls play or shop. He evaluates the importance of the day and we evaluate the need for the time away. Have we been off and running or just staying at home? There are times when I have heard that the fibro sufferer refuses to get up. They stay in bed and focus on the pain, not even knowing they are doing more harm than good for themselves! These are the times to plan small outings. Plan a trip to the porch with strawberry lemonade or a dinner on the patio. For some it may be a trip to a park bench. Distraction is fibro's saving grace! The pain is temporarily forgotten or at least ebbed. Keep planning. But stay open for change.

Our Part

It takes many parts to make a whole. We danced into our relationship with our spouse full of hopes and dreams. Illness was probably not a part of the dreams but it is a part of the reality. I have told my girls, "You will know it's love if you are willing to hold their head when they have the flu." It's true, but we would rather not test it.

We love a great piece of advice and we are willing to offer advice to others. What if there isn't any advice to be found? That's where we are, as spouses of fibro. It is our responsibility to research the options to a better life for our families.

Exercise

"Exercise is one of the most effective treatments for fibromyalgia; it alleviates all of the symptoms of fibromyalgia, including pain, fatigue, and sleep problems."[32] We all know how important exercise is, but we don't realize how hard it is to become enthusiastic when you are in pain. Imagine getting over the flu. Your body aches all over but the fever and sickness are gone. That is how it feels to a person with fibro. Now try to imagine craving a desire to work out.

Motivation for exercise is hard to find in someone with fibro. Starting out small, 5 or 10 minute walks around the block, at a mall, or around the yard are good starts. We, as the encourager, need to keep encouraging! We don't necessarily have to be present for the exercise, but it is much more fun and beneficial for the sufferer if they have someone to share the time with. Increasing the walks to 20 or 30 minutes, 3 to 5 times a week is optimal for pain management. Weight lifting, aerobics and cardio workouts depend on the fibro patient's pain tolerance. To them "No pain, no gain" means much pain and no gain. Go slow but go!

Healthy Eating Habits

Encouraging good eating habits is hard to do when lasagna and potatoes taste so good. However, there are countless easy recipes for the healthy eater that are not tasteless! "What to eat and not eat" in the fibro world is in debate. My husband's current doctor told him not to eat red meats, potatoes, and dairy and to eat nuts and whole wheat products. But recently on a television program, my husband saw a clip that stated one with fibro should not indulge in nuts, whole wheat, and dairy. The only corresponding advice I have found that everyone agrees upon is stocking up on fresh fruits and vegetables. They also agree that avoiding preservatives, high fructose corn syrup and hydrogenated oils, and white flour and white sugar as much as possible, is essential. Several studies have been done on fake sweeteners too. None of them came out good for healthy living.

One very common sweetener is "Nutrasweet" (Aspartame). The chemical make-up of this product breaks down into methanol (wood alcohol) when digested. Methanol quickly converts to formaldehyde in the body. Formaldehyde causes gradual and eventually severe damage to the neurological system, and immune system and causes permanent genetic damage at extremely low doses.[33] And the beverage industry pours this out to us by the gallons.

On the positive sweetener side, there is a plant called Stevia (*Stevia rebaudiana*),[34] producing leaves that are harvested and dried, that has been used for millennia. The naturally grown Stevia plant from South America is extremely sweet and comes with a faint flavor when used raw and is a great alternative to low or no-calorie sweetners.[35]

An important fact to understand about our digestive system is that it identifies foods that are in their purest form, knowing how to break them down and utilize them most efficiently throughout the body. The more food is processed, altered, and changed, the less the system knows how to use it. In some cases processed food and chemicals will stay in the system for long periods of time while it tries to figure out how to use it, store it, our get rid of it. The purer the food, the more useful it is and the better our body functions.

We all need cell regeneration for survival. Our bodies are created to do this automatically. Imagine if you put Jell-O in a pitcher and try to pour it like a beverage, it wouldn't pour well or be very drinkable. Fibro patients have a system that is slower, to regenerate cell growth due to lack of sleep, fatigue and stress. Their system has "slowed" down. What they eat is more important now than ever before. As the spouse, I am looking for better, healthier and easier meals to prepare at home. We seldom go out and never drink diet soda. We are also converting to a greater fruit and vegetable-portioned plate over meat and grain. I say converting because it is a slow process for us. I know for my family a sudden change in diet would cause frustration and stress.

Many fibro sufferers have multiple health conditions. Many have auto-immune issues that hinder healing and recovery from injury or illness. Our immune system can fight off viruses and illness much faster with less stress and when fed healthy foods that the body can quickly identify and distribute for expedited healing.

Water

When we built our house, we were given a "basic" appliance package. We decided to upgrade to a more "efficient" package. More water and energy efficiency appeared to be a great choice. I now know the word efficient means "an extra rinse, an extra spin, or more time to dry." We are not sure how "efficient" the appliances really are now but at least I'm not washing by hand.

With our dishwasher, when you put plates with extra junk on them, they come out dirty. I either have to rinse the dishes before putting them in the machine, or they go through an extra rinse at the end.

Our bodies are made of 80 percent water. Much like the dishwasher, if we put a lot of junk in it and not enough water, our bodies get clogged up. Most fibro sufferers take pain and sleep medications. If your spouse is not drinking enough water the medicine can remain stored up in the body for no reason and with no way to be disposed. Encouraging water drinking will help them flush out the remaining toxins left behind in their system, allowing cells to regenerate easier and oxygen to flow freer in the system.

Increased water intake can also help with irritable bowel syndrome and weight loss as well. For us, the caregivers, increased water helps our bodies function more efficiently too. No extra rinses or spin cycle needed.

Depression

There are so many days that go by that I do not think about Brent's fibro. I think about healthy eating, taking a walk, and keeping the house at a low roar but seldom his fibro. It is no wonder then that I cannot fathom his state of mind being in pain almost every waking minute. I silently wonder how he keeps from being depressed. Depression is a factor in fibro sufferers. Do they get depressed from the pain of fibro or did they have depression first? Studies show that not all fibro sufferers have depression. Some of the pain medications prescribed however, are anti-depressant, so if they were to become depressed, I guess that's serving double duty.

Over a lifetime, as many as 90 percent of fibromyalgia patients may experience symptoms of depression, and 62 percent may experience major depressive disorder.[36]

Depression and anxiety might not be present today, but it could be in the future. We as the caregivers need to be attentive to the signs of depression. If symptoms are severe enough to seek help, we need to be able to encourage professional support. It is humbling enough to be in pain but adding depression and anxiety brings an additional struggle.

In the field of psychology, there are many avenues to take to alleviate depression. There is no need to suffer for an extended period of time.

I believe when we are born we are painted into the most beautiful painting, painted specifically for each one of us! Sadly, when I get into my down times I see a blemish on my painting, a spitball of sorts. Recently I got really frustrated with the lack of ease in my life. It felt like I was swimming upstream. While talking with my youngest I realized that I really do have a nice life. I had a roof over my head, food on my table, a secure job for my husband, and two healthy, smart girls. Why was I complaining? I was focusing on that ugly spitball and not on the big picture of life. All the beauty was being ignored for one small blemish. My daughter said, "Mom, you need to look at the whole picture, brush off the spitball and move on." Wisdom from youthful thoughts!

Depression does not just affect the fibro sufferer. We, too, are human. There is reason to feel sadness about losing a dream. We had dreams to fulfill with our spouse in the future and now some of them may have to be eliminated or at best altered. The death of a dream is sad and can be depressing. However, it doesn't have to take over. There are opportunities to grow from change. A bigger picture needs to be kept in mind. Do not focus on the little pieces of disappointment but the bigger moments of beauty.

Self-care

A very large part of helping others is caring for the self. If you cannot take care of you, how will you care for others? It is important to get a good night's sleep, healthy food, plenty of water and quiet time.

Getting a full uninterrupted night's sleep of around 8 hours is optimal for health. Your body regenerates healthy cells during sleep. It fights bacteria and viruses, as well as heals while sleeping. A full night of sleep can keep one from irritability, irrational thinking, stress, and anxiety.[37] Your body digests food better when fully rested. It reacts in stressful situations more effectively and makes more efficient decisions.

Obviously, good eating habits and water help the body stay healthy. Good food can clear our skin, shine our hair, and help our nails grow strong. Great food can brighten our day, make us look forward to our next meal, and discourage binge eating and cravings. When we eat well, we feel well. When we feel well, we treat others and ourselves better. There is no guilt in eating healthfully.

When we feel good, are well fed, and rested, we have cared for the mind and body. The spirit is next. Peace and quiet are essential for keeping the physical and emotional being calm. Reading encouraging books, meditating on life or just sitting in a quiet atmosphere are great ways to settle the inner self. Studies have actually shown meditation to cure depression more effectively and longer-lasting than expensive drugs and does not have any side effects.[38] This kind of quiet pulls all loose ends together. Quiet can bring ideas to life and questions to a conclusion. It can also give you time to look at your own life and how to become a better and a more peaceful you.

Lastly, I want to encourage you not to put yourself last. You are important to your spouse and others. If you become ill, spend time healing. If you are in need of time away find a way to achieve that. You are the only you this earth gets. You have one chance at making your mark on this round planet. No one else knows exactly what you need more than you! If you were meant to be somewhere else in your life than where you are right now, then you'd probably be there instead. You in this present moment, is the only moment you get to have just like it. Make the most of where you are right now.

The Bigger Picture

There is a very big elephant in the room, you know. Yes! He stands there waiting for you to let him outside. That elephant is perception. Brent and I recently had "the talk" about that big elephant one Saturday morning. I "thought" he was angry at me and he "thought" I was avoiding him.

Lack of communication is one of the number one reasons for divorce. Silence, avoidance, verbal outbursts and placating are all forms of poor communication. They may feel right at the moment but ultimately they create a barrier that can eventually erode a marriage and dissolve vows.[39] Distance is created quickly if you don't share your feelings or tell your partner what you are noticing.

We assumed we knew each other's emotions. After almost 25 years we thought we knew each other that well. We've been perceiving life situations for years and neither of us thought we were mistaken in our assumptions. Neither of us wanted to rock that boat yet. This pattern was rock solid and the foundation was crumbling quickly.

It was simple, really. I jumped out of bed heading straight to the kitchen for breakfast. I needed an early breakfast as I was not getting a lunch break at work that day. Brent began his normal morning routine in the bathroom. I did not understand his constant barrage of petty comments about my unusual morning routine. He thought I jumped out of bed to avoid any morning pillow talk. I thought I was being efficient. I was making breakfast for both of us after all.

Before serving breakfast I felt attacked about leaving the bedroom so quickly. I left the room to gather my thoughts and emotions. I had been spending time in prayer and meditation for several months now, and I felt clarity to my emotions would come if I stepped out of the situation. It sure did, and I was ready to hash out this reoccurring confusion.

In the peace and quiet of the home office, I asked Brent, "Are you happy?" I knew my answer. "No, I was not happy." What was his? Brent answered, "No, I am not happy." He was working up to eighty hours a week and traveling one week out of every month. He was miserable. I couldn't do a thing to fix that. He felt stuck in his job due to a salary because he had a family to support, a mortgage to pay, and over 200 people at the office that relied on him.

Here's our elephant. We live in a beautiful, big, lonely house. Brent couldn't appreciate the house, the land, the family because he felt such a huge obligation financially. I couldn't appreciate the house or family because it was lonely doing all the work at home. I actually took a job at a chocolate retailer thinking the job would be fun and maybe fill a void I hadn't yet identified in my life. It worked for the twelve hours I was in the store. Selling chocolate didn't fulfill me; it was just a way to get out of the house and be with other people. We now know why the girls didn't feel at home here either. They felt their own loss and ours as well.

Money cannot be the only motivator in a family. There was so much silent stress in our house that if we didn't make some changes soon there may be no real family left.

Brent and I hashed out our feelings in that office on that day. The comfort of a decent job that supported our lifestyle was not what living life was all about. I strongly believe we have a purpose, a meaning for living on this planet. Happiness and joy seem to be byproducts of what we DO. What if happiness and joy are supposed to be the norm and all else is to adjust around that?

In the past 30 years I have spent many hours in the office of a counselor at one point or another. Not until now did I really understand why. There are a lot of professionals who know how to advise. The ability to listen and live the truth is not always obvious. But this I know. We were not born of this time on this planet to be miserable. If you need a cheerleader, even a paid one, go get help.

I asked Brent if he wanted happiness. He did. I asked the ultimate question, "Do you want a divorce?" His tearful reply was, "No." We were caught in a vicious cycle of being unhappy. So we decided to make changes from that point on that would bring us more happiness and even joy.

The lovely two-story, two-acre, four-bedroom beauty is now for sale and the job hunt is on! Is this more stressful? I do not like selling my house. I stand in a long line of those who agree that house selling is right up there with root canals. But there is happiness!! The "foot is out the door." The stress seems to come and go. The fibro seems to do the same. I have a feeling if we look at joy as a way of living and work as a means of supplying joy then perhaps I have found my niche of happiness. Brent is also getting creative in his job hunt. What would bring him joy? I too am breaking ground on new and exciting possibilities for my life.

What would bring you joy? What is stopping you? Time to clear out the room of that pesky elephant; he's taking up too much joy!

Everyone has a story of a situation that created an outcome in their life they would like to alter. No one is perfect. My parents were not perfect and they had a daughter who is not a perfect parent. I admit all this to be true. Now, what to do with it? A few options are: ignore it, acknowledge it, use it as an excuse, or use it for growth.

I had a common farm girl upbringing I thought. When one carries the past like a wet rug dragging behind them, it can be a heavy burden. I could have kept the abuse bottled up, blamed the abuser, blamed anyone who wronged me, got angry at every relationship conflict and not known what was a healthy relationship. I could have been an overbearing mom who hovered and smothered my kids. I could have drunk away my frustrations. Looking at the world through the bottom of a bottle to obscure your vantage point is a way to avoid reality. Sure, this was possible. They are however learning tools. I no longer feel a victim. I am stronger for the experiences I have faced. But I found truth, although painful for a period of time, was a much more comfortable way to live.

We are all dysfunctional to some degree but to ignore it can fester into nasty behavioral and even physical conditions. In

some healing professions the behavioral influences on the physical body are the core issues to "dis-ease". The lack of ease or harmony within the body can and does create physical ailments.[40]
Brent's family was never well-to-do. I don't know if it was important to them. The point of focus is that it created in my husband a strong desire to have more financial comfort than what he experienced as a child. He wanted to give the girls material items which weren't provided for him. That was attractive to me as well. I celebrated in the financial advantages he provided for us, not realizing that there was an underlying situation forming.

When Brent was about 12 he had a brother who became very sick. The prognosis was not good and the illness sadly lasted off and on for 30 plus years. When his brother had an episode, Brent felt he was on his own for his personal care. It soon became clear that if he needed anything, he had to excel excessively for attention or rely on himself. Both of which he carried into adulthood.

We, together, developed a financially safe and abundant life for our family. We also taught the girls that in order to have what we had there were sacrifices that some families would consider excessive. Looking back, the many hours of work Brent put in, the home upkeep, the many hours feeling like a single parent were not conducive to developing a healthy family. No one is perfect thank goodness. We all have areas in which to grow.

Looking back as a child I needed security and did not want to rock the boat. We were a bi-yearly paid farm family and I thought we were rather poor. Actually we were more financially stable than I ever felt. The boat-rocker in my family got a good deal of discipline for opening their mouth. I'm sure Brent had many feelings he was repressing as well. I see my growth. I regret not correcting the situations at a very early stage in our marriage. To my defense, I didn't know they were issues at first. Personal dysfunction keeps a person blind until they want to open their eyes. I am sure there are still issues floating around in my subconscious that are still affecting me but they will be resolved eventually.

In Brent's defense, it is the same. He didn't know there were dysfunctional issues at first. I do not regret marrying the person Brent was so many years ago. He was safe, kind, and ambitious. We have grown a lot in the past several years, sometimes together and sometimes apart. Brent is not one to analyze his short comings unless it is work-related. I do not regret our relationship or its lessons, but it has been very hard for Brent to see dysfunction of the past. In fact, it has taken many years to even acknowledge them and will take many more if not the rest of his life to grow beyond and above some of them. Aren't we all a work in progress?

Each of us has a story and it is nothing to point a finger at or place blame on. No one comes through this life clean and unscathed. What fun would it be if we weren't challenged a little here and there? However, I'm sure there are a few out there thinking the quote, "God only gives us what we can handle. I only wish He didn't think I could handle so much!" But these are your stories. Fibro is part of that story. Living as a family member or friend to someone in pain actually can provide a lesson of growth.

You are not alone in this struggle. There are so many of us out there. Here is the lesson I see. We are a special group with an amazing ability to have patience toward others and we have great compassion. Even if we are a silent, unknown number we can still influence others. We can show people that there is life with fibro and we can live a happy and albeit altered life with limited stress. We can still find joy.

We live in a global world. There are billions of people on this little orb circling the sun. There are generations upon generations of humans that have lived life here as well. Why, after millenniums, are there still so many unhappy people suffering with stress-related disorders like fibro? I ask the question and have no answer. But I am going to change my little corner, focusing on happiness and life giving joy.

My hope is that if I find my happy place and you see it then you too will find yours and you can pass it along. If you find yours first, let the rest of the world know. Reflect your joy for potential students watching you. You give, others receive, and you receive in return. We are all in this together.

Spiritual Side

I am a big believer in God. He put me here for a reason at this very time and place. I am not a mistake. My place on this planet is exactly where I am supposed to be. I have chosen the paths I walk. When the going gets tough I need to ask, "What can I learn from this?" not "Why me?" When we look to God for resolution in times of difficulty, we are going to find answers not more questions.

God did not give the world fibromyalgia. Men and women live in a stress-filled society with little direction in how to deal with the stress. We become demanding, controlling, and selfish with our time and lack introspection. When we pause and take an intentional breath we gain the ability to listen to what our bodies are asking of us. Often these situations creep up on us quietly. Without warning we enter into chaos and attempt to function at full speed, thinking that it is normal and without repercussions.

I believe my spirit belongs to God. He is the owner; I am the recipient. When we find ourselves in pain I believe it is a warning sign or a signal that we are ignoring our spiritual purpose. These physical discomforts are a way to tell us to slow down and can guide us to a different path if we are open to listening. If we ignore this 'dis-ease' within us, the pain will continue to grow. Some may believe that they can "never" heal. God can do all things and He can heal. Eventually, when we become aware of and change our self-destructive behaviors, the pain can dissipate and even heal.

The "ah-ha" moments happen when we have learned to listen to the Spirit or small voice within. The path looks much different when we turn around and look back. Hind sight, I believe all growth is good even though sometimes it is not comfortable and may even be painful. You are not alone. God walks with us and in us, showing compassion and love even in our hardest times. Some situations are not for our growth but for someone else's growth. However it is evaluated, it is growth and growth is good. God creates a stronger, more loving, and more compassionate being with growth.

This is not to say that all people choose to take their "warning sign" as growth. Some choose to remain in the condition because the fear of change is far too great. We are not attached to their condition. They may stay for a while then grow or just remain there forever. We can still love them but we need to continue on our personal path of growth.

Fibromyalgia is a tool for growth. It slows a person down. It changes a person's direction. It makes them grow. I know it is a big stretch to think fibro might actually have a positive aspect. How could anything so terrible and painful be positive? It does make one evaluate the business of their life. It will create a desire for quiet time. Fibro encourages a person to take care of oneself. It is so important to look at the silver lining. There is life on the other side of the storm.

When I was being prepped, many years ago, before brain surgery, I was asked by the doctor, "Do you want your husband to stay in the waiting room until you come out of recovery?" I knew the surgery was going to take over two hours and our girls needed him home more than I needed him waiting, so I sent him home. But that question created an acknowledgement within me that was by far larger and longer lasting than the simple words spoken. I realized I was standing at my last day's door. I could die on the operating table. It became so incredibly important for me to ask God to forgive me for all the selfish and unkind acts I had done to other people throughout my life. Please, forgive me. I also wanted to clear the air of those who had been unkind to me and let God know I had forgiven them. If I did not wake up in the morning I felt prepared to leave this earth; however, if I did wake up, I wanted a whole new start. I needed to begin anew.

Every day is an opportunity to learn to love and an opportunity to forgive and ask for forgiveness. When we hold onto anger and resentment we are hurting ourselves most. Yes, others may feel our absence or hear our sharp words but ultimately we are damaging our self-worth. Do not let fear keep you angry. Hurting others because you do not know or believe happiness exists after forgiving can be a destructive behavioral pattern. There is no advantage whatsoever to holding onto anger.

There can be a great burden felt when caring for someone always in pain. Again, it is not our pain. Letting go of the burdensome feelings and rejoicing in the opportunity to be present to love the fibro person is freeing. Burdens bring guilt and guilt brings uncomfortable feelings of disappointment and resentment. Eliminate these negative feelings as soon as they enter the mind. They will not bring you joy.

We have been given a great opportunity in this life to abandon fear and embrace the journey. When we realize that fibromyalgia has not been done to us but rather exists around us, it is easier to let go of the fear of the future "what if's" and step into the future with happiness and joy. Progress happens when we open ourselves up to change and growth. The more joy and happiness we bring into our lives the more it will grow and expand into other's lives. We do not want to miss the little moments of happiness God sprinkles into our lives. So many little pieces of forgotten pleasures have escaped our recognition until now. Be grateful for the little moments of joy, and they will expand into a greater lifetime of happiness. At first it may be a conscious effort to see them, but quickly it becomes a habit. Seeing joy and spreading happiness is contagious, even to someone with fibro.

We do not know the time or place we will be taken from this earth, but we can choose how happy we are between here and there. Today, this very minute, chose to be happy. Chose to love those around you whether you are with them or taking time away for healing yourself. Life is a choice. Make a decision and live up to it. God is waiting to brighten your journey with His sprinkles of joy along the way.

Where to from Here

As I look back on the many years my husband has had fibro I can see the points of growth. He has become gentler, more compassionate, less demanding, and softer, with gentler communicating skills. All aspects of his life have been touched by fibro. Will he continue to change? I would imagine so. I don't see why not. God's not finished with him yet!

Fibro has also become a tool for me. I find there are so many others out there with fibro, chronic pain and depression. I have compassion for them. I understand them better now than ever before.

Do I see God working in my life? Without a doubt! I have become more focused on my purpose. Do I know where this growth is going? Not a bit. There are times when I encourage it with studies and prayer. But, mostly I am just riding out the wave of growth and I'll see where it takes me. I do find my stress level depleted and my joy increased. I find peace in not always knowing the outcome. I do not need to control where I am going or resolve where I've been. I also don't encourage Brent to control life either.

We try to control life because we don't want to deal with something we are not prepared for. We do not want to do more than we can handle. I know my pace is much slower that Brent's. It is important to remain true to self. This is my pace it makes me happy and I find in it peace and satisfaction. As Brent grows, he is accepting a different pace as well. As we change so does our relationship. We are growing together on separate fulfilling journeys. No different for the girls. They too are set in their own paths. We can encourage them, but we don't want to change them. In the big picture, does getting that one project done sooner with all the stress really change the world? It is time to reevaluate our priorities and outcomes. What is important? Neither the bigger home, greater paycheck, newer car, nor brand-name clothes will bring you peace. They will only bring you a desire for a more stuff. A satisfaction of self, a true appreciation of the uniqueness one brings to this earth is where happiness begins. Yes, a roof over your head and food on the table along with a safe environment are essential to physical health. But greater than these are to love and be loved, creating a more stress-free and truly healthy life.

Brent and I are reevaluating our lives. Where would we be most happy? How much income would it really take? What career change would create the ultimate job bringing self-fulfillment and joy? We are not adding stress by dreaming, but one day we'd like to make these dreams a reality. Brent would love to own a business of some sort, write, and quilt. I love art. I'm an artist to the core. One day I will paint and draw with abandon! Until then, we will make the best of what comes our way. Make lemons into lemonade and dodge any spit balls that may be flung at our life's masterpiece.

We are all on a journey. Some of us will cross paths for a moment, others for a while, and yet others for a lifetime. I know that we only get one journey in this life. Regardless of the path, it is ours and ours alone. We are solely responsible for the outcome of our journey. Fibromyalgia has blessed my journey with personal growth, patience, and knowledge. I am learning more about myself and my husband daily. But mostly, I am learning how to appreciate my journey and be happy. Finally, when I return to God for eternity, I want Him to say "Well done, my good and faithful servant."

Brent's Note

One morning, cereal. The next day, cancer.

Those are the opening words to a poem by Richard Solly – a poem that speaks about death. The fact is that before we take our infamous last breath, we encounter many times in our life when our breath is taken away – mini deaths, if you will. When our dreams are shattered, our hopes are crushed, our expectations of the future scattered in pieces. One day everything is just as we would have it and the next day we find ourselves searching for answers, support, and the arms of embracing love.

Our journey has not been different than yours. Ours has been a journey of searching, finding, losing again, and always adjusting to the "new normal." One would think that after writing two books on fibromyalgia and living with it for

16 years that we would have adjusted for better or worse to what life provided. So, you can imagine my trepidation when Tina revealed that she wrote a new book on fibro and our relationship. You can further imagine my hesitancy when I heard, "You may not like everything I said."

What you have before you, however, is the most transparent, real, and honest revealing of our lives. You get to hear what is real in marriage and although everything often looks packaged like a gift with a bow, there are true struggles, disagreements, and frustration along the way. Love knows no bounds. There are times of great joy and times of inner and outer conflict. There are hearts, flowers, and candy on Valentine's Day and tears, anger, and disappointment on Sweetest Day (well, maybe only once because I didn't know the rule about buying appliances).

We celebrated our 25th wedding anniversary this year because we were and are committed to each other and to the words in our vows – for better or worse. Of course, we had no idea what they meant then and may not have signed up for the gig if someone had explained it to us in detail. But, that is what life is about. Who really wants to know what lies ahead? Do you really want to anticipate for years knowing that a life changing event is going to happen to you in two years on June 1st? Or, who of us wants to know the anniversary date of our own death? God designed life in such a way as to allow us to change, to grow, and to continually love. We stumble, we fall, and we manage to get back up again – sometimes slowly and sometimes very slowly, but hopefully you have at least one other person you can turn to who will reach down and grab you by the hand, pull you up, dust you off, and wipe away the embarrassment.

Life is about living. It's about the bumps and the bruises and the agonies of defeat but more importantly it's about who we become along the way. I am certainly not the same person that I was when I first got diagnosed with fibromyalgia and hopefully, I'm not the same person you just read about. Every day I attempt to be better than I was yesterday. I don't have any regrets though of course; I could have done some things differently along the way. What I know now is that we pass down our dysfunction and our characteristics to our next generation and the generation after that. We need to break the cycles of pain and disappointment, our maladjustments and malfunctions so that our grandchildren and their children do not grow up with the hurt of our lives. There is still time! There is hope for the future! *There is still hope for me!*

I certainly hope that you have enjoyed this wonderful work of art – this interweaving of our lives as honestly as we could have portrayed them and when you see us on the street, please do not look at a neatly wrapped present with a bow. Instead, look at two humans trying to find their way in the world, a way of growth and learning that brings us to eternity, to a God that we know and love. Thank you for sharing this part of your lives with us. And, ultimately, thank you to my wonderful wife who had the courage day after day to work through issues to support and challenge us and get to the heart of the puzzle.

Now, off to get some ice cream!

Love, Brent

Stephanie's Note

When I was first asked to write this letter I didn't know what to say. Not because I did not want to write, I was honored when asked. But because for me as a child it wasn't, "My dad has fibro." He did and that changed some things, but he was still my dad. It was no separate entity inflicting my father. It wasn't him, the real him, one day and fibro dad the next. As a little girl there was no differentiation.

If Fibromyalgia taught me anything it was to alter my expectations. I expected to still run full speed into daddy with a hug when he walked in the door after work. I had to learn gentleness. I expected him to play volleyball in the backyard. I had to learn patience while he watched me with a keen eye to critique. I also expected him to help me tack up my horse in the dead of winter only to watch him run to the heated viewing room instead. Here, I learned grace and independence too.

I don't intend to make my dad sound debilitating and ill. We still went to waterparks and ran straight for knee surfing and the "toilet bowl" ride nearly every summer. We went to baseball games where he taught me how to keep score and he came to every marching band competition helping us late into the night. There were special planned daddy-daughter date days when mom escaped for a weekend away, and so much more. I guess what I am saying is I don't feel like I missed out.

I give a lot of credit to him for fighting through the hard days and the days my sister and I were not so perfect at understanding. But I give a lot of credit to my mom too. She was proactive from day one hearing his diagnosis. This was not going to break her family. She did just as you are doing now, reading, researching, and loving. You my dear friend are helping beyond words. In case you haven't heard it yet, "Thank you." May you be blessed with patience, mercy, and grace. May you find strength when you need it, tears to help heal, and the wisdom to face Fibromyalgia without defeat. My heart and love go out to you.

Love, Stephanie

Alexis' Note

The happiest memories I have with my dad were always made on vacation. I remember his smile and laugh after sliding down a crazy waterslide at the Kalahari Resort in Wisconsin Dells. To me, living with someone who suffers from Fibromyalgia is almost like living around one who struggles with a mental illness. I did not understand my dad's pain, all I wanted to do was take it away and make his life happy again. The pain is more than physical it is a psychological reminder of what one cannot control. This disease eats away at your health, energy and happiness. Overtime when one focuses on someone else's pain you can begin to take it on as your own. You take on the habits of a cautious control freak, scared of the outside world.

When I was young I feel I grew up completely oblivious from the outside world because of a struggle both of my parents had trying to find safety in dad's unexplainable pain and suffering. My dad's smile began to fade when he began to suffer from fibro and I rarely saw that smile in a regular life setting. The pain was in every part of his life. It was as though a cloud was always hiding the sun, like one who suffers from depression or mental angst; similar emotional patterns are seen in someone whom suffers with physical pain.

My mom sees it differently than I do. Plain and simple, my sister and I were very sheltered from society up until high school. We were in a parochial school and on a small farm that did not give us much social interaction. Now that we have grown up and moved out we realize how the crosses we bare have roots deeper than we know. We see these challenges and struggles through rose-colored glasses. They will always be much more complicated to handle than expected.

Recently my mom and I were discussing my unease with social anxiety. She admitted to having some of the same feelings with a few differences. I never knew she had anxiety about being in social situations! I always thought she was strong and resilient to anxiety. Socially challenged by the same stresses she, my sister and myself all suffer from a sort of social anxiety or an over sensitivity leading to becoming easily overwhelmed in situations. None of us had expressed these dysfunctions over the years. I don't think we knew they were dysfunctions until we saw what the norm was outside our small family environment. I can see how this happens. We learned these behaviors as a family, feeling each other's energy of pain, confusion and misunderstanding. My dad dealt with his pain behind closed doors trying to hide it as much as possible and never shared it outside our family unit. We all learned how to push aside painful issues and ignore them even if it meant increasing personal stress and the unknown dysfunction.

There is a problem that arises when pain is packed away. It builds up like a volcano waiting to erupt. I've seen my dad "blow" expressing all the built up anger from weeks or months in one explosion. I've seen my sister follow in those footsteps as well and at times my mom and I too. When I realized releasing it all at once was hurting those around me and was a bad solution, I fell back into suppressing my feelings. The anger and sadness gets released in other not so pleasant ways I have found. Acne, stomachaches and particularly "dis-ease" like physical pain and sickness are attributed to repressed feelings. This endless cycle overtime just continues to get worse and I saw this in my own life to the point that I was going to be like my dad if I didn't make some changes. My dad too has begun to see this in his own life as medication, dieting and exercise still do not resolve all of his pain.

I put off writing this letter for months. Seriously, multiple months I even had to walk away from it completely and return to it a month later. Wounds don't heal over-night. The crosses we bare won't go away in a blink of an eye. Please don't think I had a horrible and unloving childhood. My parents loved me very much. There were times of great joy and as my mom says, I do love to stop and smell the roses. All of these experiences are part of my personal development. They make up who I am today and I am growing to love this person I am becoming. The same patterns I struggled with growing up I still struggle with today. I put this letter off because I was putting off facing the pain and the growth. When my mom came to me and told me she was writing a book about living with Fibro I was confused as to why. To me, all the pain I dealt with for the past 15 plus years had been suppressed enough that I could move forward and learn from it rather than it hurting me. I did not understand why my mom would want to bring up that pain all over again. After writing this letter and going through a few months of emotional cleansing I realized this book is her way of healing and growing from the pain. Suppressing emotions help very little. The same dysfunctional habits will continue to be repeated if depression, stress and anxiety are not faced head on.

My mom came to me and asked me to work out the pain I have ignored for so long and for that I thank her. I have let go of the pain and used it to grow, learn and change. Most importantly I learned to love my dad for who he is, not for what his fibro makes him. He is still growing and learning every day like me. My dad still has his bad days but that's okay, that doesn't impact me negatively anymore. I have learned that through my joy whether he feels joyous or not I can share and spread my love. I can encourage him to get out and spend time with the family and I can be the example of the joy and love that is lost in the pain. I can go smell the roses, spend time appreciating a moment of doing nothing in particular and feel no guilt. You can't change them just as you can't change an addict, one who has a mental illness, or one with physical pain. No matter how much you want to make them see a better way of life, you must accept them and love them for who they are. Being who you truly and joyfully are, an example of God's love is the hope to be an example they will see and want to repeat.

Moving forward I hope to live a more open and stress free life, one with less angst and sadness, fewer clouds and more sun. I hope to spread more joy and truth about life. Living is not easy but the rewards are great and abundant. I do not think my past was a mistake but perhaps the way I was looking at it was. My past was my catapult to who I am today and who I will become tomorrow. Fibromyalgia is a part of my past and I contribute it to be a large part of who I love in myself today.

With love, Alexis

Epilogue

Developing a goal for the future was not really a topic of conversation in my childhood home. We were farmers and trusted that once the crops were planted, the rains would come, and the crops would grow and one day be harvested. The fertilizer was spread at a set time every year. Crop rotation happened on an expected pattern. There wasn't really a need for building goals except to further the farm. Interruptions from Mother Nature on the farm were accepted as though they were an everyday topic of conversation. Some days they were. Was there enough rain? Was there going to be an early frost? Had the drought harmed the overall harvest?

Fibromyalgia can feel like a drought without much hope for rain. Brent and I have seen our fair share of drought, shallow communication, tough days of understanding, and what felt like endless days of just existing. We went through the questions that could end our marriage or help us continue our life together. We wanted to make goals for the future, but with Fibromyalgia living in our house it seemed futile. Tomorrow was not a guarantee. We did not know if the continued pain would increase or dissipate. Did we dare hope?

There have been marked improvements in Brent's health over the past year! After his hernia surgery and the statin mix-up, he has adapted to a different eating style hopefully eliminating the cholesterol medication all together. I was given the green light to experiment with my meal preparation. I have researched what foods cause inflammation and complications with the symptoms Brent struggles with. There is also a list of foods that create healing and well-being in the body. These have become a focus in my meal preparation and pain elimination.

Whatever it is we have been doing is working! I cannot take all the credit. Now that we are no longer attached to a large mortgage and have down-sized our possessions and living space, Brent has found more peace and calm. We are spending more time together and communication is actually more honest.

We have begun to dream! He is going back to school for a Master's degree and I am focusing my spare time on

drawing, painting, and writing. We both have lifestyles that are giving us joy together and individually.
Where is Brent's Fibromyalgia? It is almost nonexistent! He does have small bouts of pain here and there but it is not a focus of his everyday life. Usually, the increase of pain comes with the increase of stress from work or family. We have set goals to eliminate the stressors and increase joyful times and peace in our lifestyle which is working.

Where is the ice cream and lasagna? Sadly it is in Brent's vocabulary more than it is on his plate, but to be pain-free, we'll take that! I make meals of vegetables, fruit, and lean meats. Seldom do we have carbohydrates and when I do incorporate them it is usually a wild rice or colored potato. There are very few sugary snacks but a lot more fruits, flavorful teas and fruit smoothies. Even when he travels he sticks to the new eating habits.

He still gets his required sleep and uses a fragrant array of essential oils before going to bed. Additionally, however, he has added essential oils in his daily life. The medicine cabinet looks different now too. He is down to only a few prescription drugs and is hopeful to eliminate more in the near future. The vitamin store gets our hard-earned money not the pharmacy now. There is a great deal of research that goes into making a decision of what vitamin to purchase, because there is a lot of processed nonsense out there and vitamins and oils can be rather costly.

Where are we going from here? Good question! We are making plans and setting goals. We are happier with our daily lives than we have been in so many years! My silent prayer is that it continues to progress in the direction it has been going.

I have intentions to continuing this research for all of the caregivers, spouses, and friends who are caring for a loved one with Fibromyalgia. Fibromyalgia is not nice nor is it consistent but there are patterns that cannot be ignored. Some symptoms are common and some behaviors are typical to one who has fibro. There must be a code to crack in the world of pain to eliminate this cycle of discomfort for everyone.

Like the farmer who plants the seed and lets God whisper over it, "Grow," I too am planting a seed. Now I will let God take the lead and teach me in the ways I must go. There will be a harvest and it will be beautiful and pain free!

Acknowledgements

Without my life experiences Married to Fibro would be an ordinary book of medical information. First on my list of gratitude is my Creator, God. He has blessed me with a second chance at life, the opportunity to be a mother, wife, sister, Nana and friend.

A big thank you to my husband for gracefully accepting the unloading of intimate details of our marriage and friendship in this piece of literature I have often called therapy.

To my girls, big hugs of appreciation for all of the life experiences you have given me that have taught me so much.

There are several girlfriends who have experienced my walk living with Fibromyalgia in my home from the very beginning and those friends who have entered in on the way, your friendship is invaluable.

A big shout out to all of you who had input in the making of Married to Fibro, every thought created a response and improvement to this work. Those at National Fibromyalgia Association; http://www.fmaware.org/, in Self-Publishing School; https://self-publishingschool.com/, and social media have been awesome!

Finally, but never last, my siblings, parents, relatives, and all who have touched my life making me who I am today and all those days leading up to now, I am a member of an awesome family. As you read and find something changing you, thank you! Making this world a little better, even if one person at a time, fills my spirit with joy and gratitude.

For you my readers, a special thank you! You are fabulous caregivers and friends!

I welcome comments and thoughts about Married to Fibro at Marriedtofibro@yahoo.com

References

1. http://www.adaa.org/understanding-anxiety/related-illnesses/other-related-conditions/fibromyalgia

2. http://www.webmd.com/fibromyalgia/guide/fibromyalgia-and-depression

3. http://www.niams.nih.gov/health_info/fibromyalgia/

4. http://www.prohealth.com/library/showarticle.cfm?libid=8931

5. https://sleepfoundation.org/sleep-disorders-problems/fibromyalgia-and-sleep

6. http://www.health.com/health/gallery/0,,20345635,00.html

7. http://forums.webmd.com/3/fibromyalgia-exchange/forum/5824

8. http://www.orthop.washington.edu/?q=patient-care/articles/arthritis/fibromyalgia.html

9. http://www.mayoclinic.org/healthy-lifestyle/adult-health/in-depth/sleep/art-20048379

10. http://www.cnn.com/2008/HEALTH/conditions/07/14/hm.fibromyalgia/index.html?eref=rss_latest

11. http://www.mayoclinic.org/diseases-conditions/fibromyalgia/expert-answers/is-fibromyalgia-hereditary/faq-20058091

12. http://examinedexistence.com/type-a-vs-type-b-personality-traits-similiarities-and-differences/

13. http://www.2knowmyself.com/Type_A_personality_definition_characteristics_traits/what_is_a_type_a_personality_behaviour_stress

14. http://www.huffingtonpost.com/2014/01/13/are-you-a-type-a-or-type-_n_4549312.html

15. http://www.smalleymarriage.com/resources/articles.php?catID=8&resID=141

16. https://www.seasalt.com/salt-101/epsom-salt-uses-benefits

17. http://www.healthcentral.com/chronic-pain/fibromyalgia-254553-5.html

18. http://www.webmd.com/drugs/2/drug-1098-1289/aleve-oral/naproxen-oral/details/list-sideeffects

19. http://www.eatthis.com/what-happens-to-your-body-when-you-eat-fast-food

20. http://www.huffingtonpost.com/2014/01/13/are-you-a-type-a-or-type-_n_4549312.html

21. http://www.webmd.com/balance/tc/healing-through-humor-topic-overview

22. http://www.arthritis.org/about-arthritis/types/fibromyalgia/articles/fibro-fog.php

23. http://www.fibromyalgia-symptoms.org/fibromyalgia_weather.html

24. http://www.nolo.com/legal-encyclopedia/will-social-security-approve-disability-benefits-fibromyalgia.html

25. http://www.everydayhealth.com/fibromyalgia/101/fibromyalgia-and-disability.aspx

26. http://www.webmd.com/fibromyalgia/guide/fibromyalgia-work-and-disability

27. http://www.webmd.com/fibromyalgia/guide/fibromyalgia-and-exercise

28. https://www.sharecare.com/health/fibromyalgialiving/how-my-relationship-be-affected-by-fibromyalgia

29. http://www.cnn.com/2009/HEALTH/12/29/chronic.pain.relationship/

30. https://womensglib.wordpress.com/2010/07/23/fibro myalgia-linked-to-increased-suicide-risk-in-tragically-ableist-article/

31. http://www.reuters.com/article/us-fibromyalgia-suicide-idUSTRE66F3JJ20100716

32. http: //www.webmd.com/fibromyalgia/fibromyalgia-pain-10/fibromyalgia-exercise-one-step-time

33. http://www.holisticmed.com/aspartame/embalm.html Aspartame (nutrasweet) breaks down into methanol (wood alcohol).28.http://www.news-medical.net/health/Fibromyalgia-Depression-and-Anxiety.aspx

34. https://en.wikipedia.org/wiki/Stevia_rebaudiana

35. https://authoritynutrition.com/stevia/

36. http://www.news-medical.net/health/Fibromyalgia-Depression-and-Anxiety.aspx

37. http://www.better-sleep-better-life.com/benefits-of-sleep.html

38. https://www.psychologytoday.com/blog/mindfulness-in-frantic-world/201110/curing-depression-mindfulness-meditation

39. http://patch.com/georgia/marietta/the-top-10-reasons-marriages-end-in-divorce_14370092

40. http://scienceblogs.com/insolence/2013/03/19/disease-dis-ease-whats-the-difference/

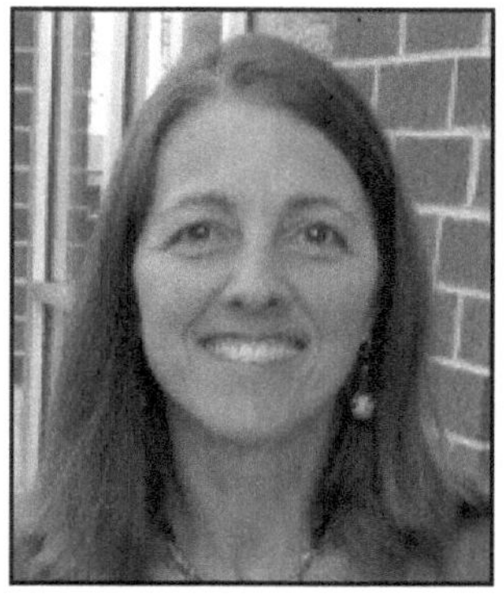

About the Author

Tina Marie Birkhoff is an artist from birth, a designer by trade and a health enthusiast at heart. She has studied at great lengths the necessity of eating, living, and praying for greater health. After having a brush with death, a scare with cancer and a husband who has been challenged with Fibromyalgia for over ten years, researching a healthy lifestyle became a necessity. Her husband is no longer suffering from the depilating characteristics of fibromyalgia thanks to her extensive research and successful application of healthy living. As a successful organic gardener and preserver her family and friends reap the benefits of great food, uplifting conversation and wholesome living.

Tina graduated from Northern Illinois University with a BFA and continues to be creative with many forms of artistic medium. Her art work has been displayed in several galleries across the Midwest, online, and can be viewed and purchased at www.TinaMarieGallery.org.

Comments are welcomed at Marriedtofibro@yahoo.com

Tina and her husband live in Prescott Arizona and return to the Midwest often to visit family and friends.

www.ingramcontent.com/pod-product-compliance
Lightning Source LLC
Chambersburg PA
CBHW050446290526
45786CB00006B/2189

* 9 7 8 1 5 3 9 3 4 6 7 4 6 *